VEGAN
OR
WE'RE GONE

Hence
^ PLANET BEFORE PALATE

Muthukumar Ramalingam

Illustrations and Cover design
Manasa M

To all our animal friends.

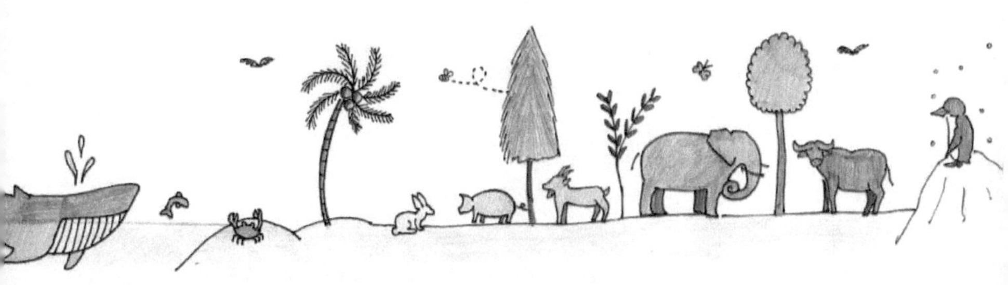

PRAISE FOR VEGAN OR WE'RE GONE

"A brilliant and a detailed overview of all things vegan. Plenty of food for thought for anyone curious about the vegan diet as well as practicing vegans. A must read. I pray for wide distribution of this informative and timely book."

Seth Tibbott
Founder and Chairman of Tofurky USA & Author

—————

"I love this book! A great, to the point, yet comprehensive, easy-to-read book that clearly explains why going vegan is so important!

Whether you've never heard about being vegan, been thinking about going vegan, or are a vegan activist - this book should be part of your collection.

It brings together a huge range of reasons to go (as the book is so appropriately titled) "Vegan or We're Gone", all in just 200 well-written and researched pages that are creatively arranged in an interesting, reader-friendly and easy to use manner."

Zac Lovas
Co-Founder of VegVoyages - Vegan Adventure Tours, USA

—————

"An excellent book. Though it speaks about a serious issue of justice, the lucid writing along with illustrations, anecdotes, quotes, and poems, keep the readers engaged. You strike the right chord at the right places. Engaging content."

FOREWORD

By Dr Rupa Shah

I am very happy to read this wonderfully engaging book "Vegan or We're Gone" by Muthu. This book will help in creating awareness about compassionate way of life.

The chapters are succinct, and each one is about an important topic regarding veganism. The chapters compel us to consider how we can change our way of being – thinking, loving, and living. The book has covered almost all aspects of the vegan lifestyle.

Veganism is about animals and is for animals. "Vegan or We're Gone" explains why we all can embrace the vegan way of life for our growth and evolution and that, animals are our fellow beings on this planet. Animals are our responsibility to look after and we have to evolve together.

The book is written in a lucid style, and the message is very powerful. One of the highlights is the beautiful artwork that is woven into the book by artist, Manasa, which lends the project with oodles of charm.

Anyone who wants to begin their vegan journey should read this book to be fully aware and inspired about why the world can be vegan.

Best Wishes,

Dr Rupa Shah, MBBS
Founder, Speaker & Author
Publisher - Compassion India Magazine

By Kuntal Joisher

I had a chance to read and review "Vegan or We're gone" by Muthu.

Quite a thorough, detailed, and a comprehensive take on several aspects around Veganism.

This book is for anyone and everyone, may it be a Non-vegetarian, or a Vegetarian, or even a Vegan - to get a better understanding of what Veganism is, how to take your first steps, and also several issues including ethics, sustainability, environment, health, fitness, and nutrition. The book is a one stop shop!

I've been a Vegan for about 18 years now, and I've climbed to the top of Mt. Everest twice so far. And so one thing that I can say without a shred of doubt is that "no animal needs to suffer or die for our dreams to come true including climbing to the top of Everest."

So go Vegan - for the animals, for the planet, and for yourself.

Kuntal Joisher
Vegan Mountaineer who scaled Mt. Everest

Contents

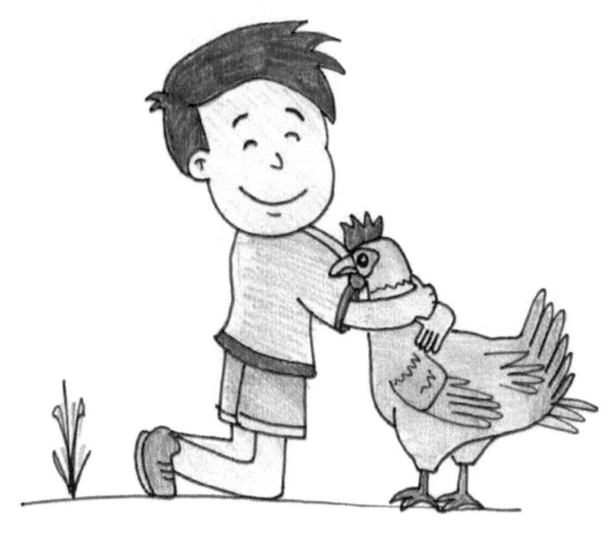

"Animals are my
friends.

And I don't eat my
friends."

George Bernard Shaw

CHAPTER 1

WARNING AND A REQUEST

Warning first: We are at a tipping point.

Billions of land animals and trillions of marine animals are killed every year, for food and human gains, causing unimaginable violence and misery to animals.

In addition to taking away the freedom and the right of animals to live their life, this immeasurable, no-end-in-sight, extra-large-scale massacre is also damaging, forever, the only home we have – planet Earth.

Farming of animals, breeding, slaughtering them for food, fishing, and hunting wildlife are the main reasons for global warming, natural calamities, species extinction, pandemics, and world hunger.

Food on our plates is the next nuclear bomb – but incorrectly labeled as meat or dairy.

It is time to discover the links between our planet, our plate, and our palate. These are more tightly linked than we can ever imagine.

It is time to stop the animal breeding and massacre. It is time to put animals and our planet before our palate.

Because either we go ***vegan or we're gone!***

Sincere Request

"We all who claim to care about the well-being of human beings and the preservation of our environment should become vegans for that reason alone.

By doing this, we would thereby increase the amount of grains and food available to feed people elsewhere who are hungry, reduce pollution, save water, save energy, and stop contributing to the clearing of forests.

Moreover, a plant-based diet is cheaper than one based on meat. It is healthy and results in reduced medical expenses. Hence, we would have more money available to devote to our family, education, flood relief, community welfare or whatever social or political cause that seems important."

– Peter Singer

Peter Albert David Singer is an Australian philosopher, Professor of Bioethics at Princeton University, and Professor at University of Melbourne. Singer is a cofounder of Animals Australia and the founder of The Life You Can Save.

CHAPTER 2

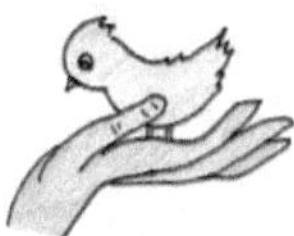

WHAT DOES IT MEAN TO BE A VEGAN?

Veganism is not a sacrifice. It is a joy.

Veganism is NOT a diet. It is not just about food. Veganism is not only about you or me.

Veganism is about them. It is about every animal's right to life. It is about stopping the exploitation of animals for our own selfish use.

Veganism is not a trend or fashion. Veganism is not a process of giving up what you like.

Veganism is about giving, that is, giving animals the life that they deserve. Veganism is also giving fellow humans their share of food and water. Veganism is giving a peaceful and compassionate world for everyone, animals and humans alike.

Veganism is a realization. It is an awakening. It is a deep understanding that other animals wish to live, just like we do, and that they have a right to do so. It is a realization that we do not have a right to take away the life of animals who do not want to die or torture them.

It is definitely a lot easier to stop consuming or using any animal products than it is to get crammed in a cage, waiting to be slaughtered.

Veganism is not always done out of love for animals. Rather it is an act of justice and an understanding that animals are individuals and that they do not exist to be exploited by us.

In the words of Mahatma Gandhi, "The greatness of a nation and its moral progress can be judged by the way its animals are treated."

"If you really care about animals, then stop trying to figure out how to exploit them 'compassionately'. Just stop exploiting them" said Gary L. Francione, Professor of Law at Rutgers University School, Newark and an animal rights advocate.

Let us repeat. Veganism is NOT a diet. It is not about food. It is not a weight loss plan. It is not about finding alternatives for meat, fish, eggs, milk, or dairy.

It is about finding ways to deliver justice to animals who cannot speak or stand up against human atrocities and annihilation.

It is about being the voice for the voiceless.

Veganism is the hardest thing to do if you look at it from your point of view. Veganism is the easiest thing to do if you look at it from the animals' point of view.

CHAPTER 3

TWO SIDES OF THE SAME COIN

Our food habits have been shaped over years by family, tradition, culture, and religion.

We are in general either a non-vegetarian or a vegetarian. But to what extent are these two food habits different?

Being a non-vegetarian is about consuming meat, eggs, and dairy, in addition to plants. Being a vegetarian is about consuming dairy, in addition to plants.

You will be surprised to know that both being a non-vegetarian or vegetarian are almost the same. They are two sides of the same coin.

Both are food habits picked up blindly over a period of time, based on tradition, religion, or family practices, without being questioned by us, of their morality.

Both meat and dairy are from animals. Non-vegetarians and vegetarians, both trouble, directly or indirectly, animals, for selfish reasons – calling it "for food or for survival or for health" so that it doesn't sound that bad.

Being a non-vegetarian is about torturing and killing of many species – chickens, goats, pigs, and cows. Being a vegetarian is mostly about troubling and torturing just one species – cows – for dairy.

Being a non-vegetarian is about instant killing of animals. Being a vegetarian is about slow killing of cows in installments – by way of artificial insemination, injecting hormones to improve milking, separating calves from the mother, and ultimately sending them to slaughterhouses.

Dairy and meat are more strongly connected than one would think. Across the globe, including India, there is no such thing as cattle raised solely for beef. Therefore, the dairy industry is the primary supplier of cattle to the beef industry. For example, in India, 90% of cows that are slaughtered for meat are from the dairy industry.

If we consume milk or dairy, we are supporting the beef industry and the slaughter of cows without we being aware of it. By buying milk, we subsidize the cost of meat. If people stop buying milk, cost of cow meat will go up by three times.

Both non-vegetarian and vegetarian ways of living are not good for animals, environment, and Mother Earth.

The age-old concept of ahimsa, or non-violence toward fellow sentient beings, has evolved into veganism, an idea that is rapidly transforming the globe, especially in the last 50 years. If you are a vegan, you eat only plant-based food and do not harm animals in any way. Vegans do not consume meat, cheese, milk, dairy, and eggs and also do not use animal products in day-to-day life.

Meat and dairy both are unnatural food choices, and we all have been forced to consume these during our years of growing up.

"We are all born vegan. World's oldest and strongest addiction is meat" says Gary Yourofsky, an eminent vegan activist based in Michigan, USA.

Fact! : You can live only on plants but you can not live only on meat or dairy. Meat for example does not contain fiber, vitamins or minerals, where is plants do. Vitamin C, crucial for immune function, collagen production, and iron absorption, vitamin A, essential for vision, immune function, and cell growth and Magnesium, important for muscle and nerve function, blood sugar control, and bone health, for example are only available in plants.

CHAPTER 4

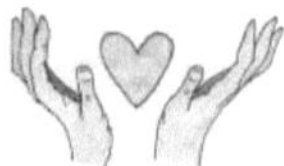

WHAT ABOUT MY HEALTH?

People eat meat thinking that they will become as strong as an ox, forgetting that the ox eats grass.

If you think a little bit, you will know that plant is the only source of all protein on earth!

Plant-based foods have protein, calcium, vitamins, and amino acids. Plant protein and plant calcium are much better for our health than animal protein or animal calcium.

According to American Dietetic Association and Dietitians of Canada, "Appropriately planned plant-based diets are healthful, nutritionally adequate, and provide health benefits in the prevention and treatment of many diseases. Well-planned vegan and other types of plant-based diets are appropriate for all stages of the life cycle, including during pregnancy, lactation, infancy, childhood, and adolescence."

Plant-based foods provide protein, fiber, and a variety of micronutrients and phytochemicals that provide protection against many diseases.

It is now a well-known fact that plant-based food reduces unwanted fats and cholesterol, reduces risk of heart and cardiovascular diseases, reduces risk of diabetes, high blood pressure, cancers, joint pains, and other chronic diseases such as muscular degeneration and cataracts.

The long-held belief that milk is high in calcium and hence is good for our bones has been proven incorrect by research.

Pasteurization and homogenization of cows' milk make the calcium contained useless. In fact, drinking processed milk is one of the main causes of osteoporosis, that is, weakening of bones. On the other hand, plant-based food such as green leafy vegetables, lady's finger, and sweet potatoes contain great amounts of calcium.

Many people consume meat and dairy saying they contain vitamin B12. But where do animals or cows get their B12 from? From gut bacteria and dirt.

Similar to cows, our gut bacteria synthesizes B12 required by our body. It is not necessary that we consume animal products to get B12. Unwashed vegetables also contain B12 and hence, a bit of dirt is okay. There are also plant-based B12 supplements in the market for those who need.

Probiotics are often referred to as good bacteria. Fermented foods that we consume as a part of our diet contain great amounts of good bacteria. In addition, there are many vegan foods that contain as much probiotics and vitamins that are found in yogurt, which are explained in detail later in this book.

Kuntal Joisher, a vegan mountaineer who climbed The Mount Everest successfully twice, says "One of the biggest myths about vegan diet is that they are nutritionally deficient because they lack protein. I wanted to dispel that myth. I climbed Mount Everest as a vegan and did so in the harshest conditions."

CHAPTER 5

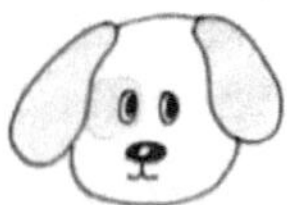

DOGS' MILK IS FOR PUPPIES

Do you know any species on earth that drink milk of another species? Weirdly enough, humans do.

Human's milk is for human babies, not for others. In the same way, cow's milk is for baby cows.

Dogs do not drink pig's milk. Pigs do not drink cow's milk. Tigers do not drink elephant milk. Elephants do not drink lion's milk. Goats do not drink human milk. But only humans drink the milk of another species!

Please remember this: Cows give milk not because they are cows. They give milk because they are "mothers". All mothers give milk. Mother's milk is for their babies, – be it humans, dogs, lions, monkeys, or cows.

Dairy industry is pure exploitation of the female reproductive system of cows.

Here are reasons why you should say no to milk, cheese, and other dairy products:

- Cows on dairy farms are repeatedly impregnated by means of artificial insemination and forced to undergo multiple pregnancies which exploits cows' reproductive system.

- Baby cows are separated from mothers at birth. Stress and fear plague these cows on a daily basis.

- Male calves are destined to become veal.

- Cows are regularly fed oxytocin hormone so that they can produce more milk. Oxytocin residues in milk causes premature puberty in females and breast enlargement in males.

- Cows are chained to milking machines, causing ulcers.

- Milk consumption is linked to many diseases such as osteoporosis, that is, bone weakening.

- Dairy cows are fed steroids, antibiotics, and even food containing animal meat.

- However differently obtained, animal fat and butter are nevertheless similar.

- When cows have nothing left to give, they are sent to a slaughterhouse.

- Animals in the dairy industry go through horrific cruelty which you can see in many YouTube videos.

- In India and elsewhere, beef industry exists only because of the dairy industry.

- In India, there is no such thing as cattle raised solely for beef. Therefore, the dairy industry is the primary supplier of cattle to the beef industry.

- If you consume milk or dairy, you are supporting the beef industry and the slaughter of animals. If you want to save cows from being killed, stop dairy.

"What I hear about milk is un-digestible." – I hear you.

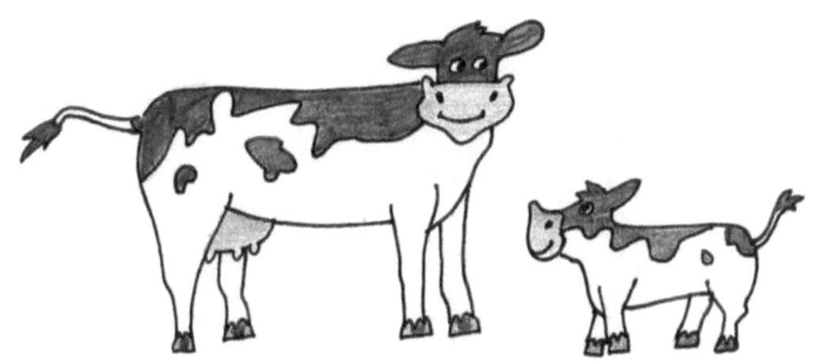

Yes. I do not drink milk.
No. I am not lactose intolerant;
I am cruelty intolerant.

Manasa
Author and animal rights activist

Dogs' milk is for puppies

CHAPTER 6

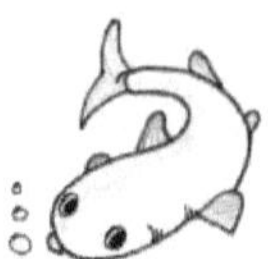

CAN I EAT FISH? YES, FOR THE NEXT 25 YEARS!

We have an option to wake-up now or wake-up after 25 years, that is, in 2050!

If we continue to do fishing the way we do now, oceans of the world will be fishless by 2050 (2048 to be precise) as per detailed research by *The Journal of Science.* Year 2050 is just 25 years away and will pass quickly.

Our freshwater and marine (ocean) environments are very fragile today and are getting damaged every day by a number of human activities including overfishing. Overfishing is catching fish faster than stocks can replenish.

Unmonitored and irresponsible fishing practices are being held as one of the major culprits behind this potential disaster.

According to an FAO report (a unit of the United Nations), global production of fish and other aquatic animals, for food, has reached close to 223 million tons in 2022. With a growing human population, this will increase further, impacting already fragile rivers and oceans.

Subsidies and support provided to the fishing industry is one of the main causes of overfishing. Such subsidies reduce production costs, which otherwise would not make any economic sense or environmental sense. The United Nations (Agenda for Sustainable Development) has called for an end to harmful subsidies of fishing and to reduce fishing itself.

In order to accomplish the goal of marine conservation, governments are thinking of implementing policies that define daily fishing limits per species, limiting the number of days at sea, putting a cap on the number of fishing boats allowed in one area, prohibiting spears and bait, setting minimum mesh sizes, and placing restrictions based on seasons.

All these would not be required, if we – you & I – implement a personal policy of being vegan in our daily life.

If we are vegan, that is, one who cares for animals, our earth, the environment, and our future generations, in a holistic way, we will not eat fish.

* * *

Fishing is cruel.

Matthieu Ricard, author of *A Plea for the Animals*, was able to look at this from the eyes of the fish:

"Suddenly I saw that whole scene in a different light: a fish pulled from its vital element by an iron hook stuck through its mouth, then suffocating in the air, the way we drown in water. In order to lure the fish to the hook, did I not also skewer (pin, split) a worm as living bait, thus sacrificing one life to destroy another?"

"How could I have let my mind block out this reality of suffering for such a long time? Sickened to the heart by these thoughts, I gave up fishing and fish on the spot"

When is our turn?

CHAPTER 7

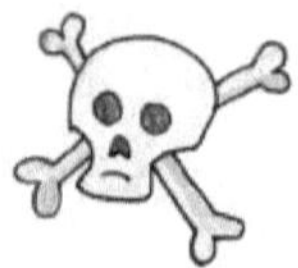

TWO WEEKS TO DIE!

By the time you finish reading this chapter, 200,000 land animals and 8,000,000 marine animals would have got killed.

If you line up all the land animals slaughtered in the United States alone in a year, you will be shocked to know that the line will come around the earth 76 times!

This is just about United States which consumes 10 billion land animals in a year. Imagine what would be the case if you add all other countries. Globally 70 billion land animals and 3 trillion marine animals are killed each year.

In the past fifty years, the number of people on the planet has doubled. The amount of meat we eat has tripled.

The amount of destruction we are causing to our co-travelers – animals – and our planet Earth is huge and enormous.

Do you know that if the human population gets killed at the rate at which we are currently killing animals for food and other needs, all of us will be gone in just two weeks?

If we include fish and marine animals, we will be gone in one day!

We kill animals for our food. We kill animals as a part of our traditions. We kill animals for our experiments, our clothing, beauty and cosmetics. We kill animals in billions each year.

"The animals of the world exist for their own reasons. They were not made for humans any more than blacks were made for whites or women for men", says Alice Walker, an American novelist and social activist.

Leonardo Da Vinci said, "The time will come when men such as I will look upon the murder of animals as they now look upon the murder of men."

The picture below shows the number of animals slaughtered for food in just 1 minute.

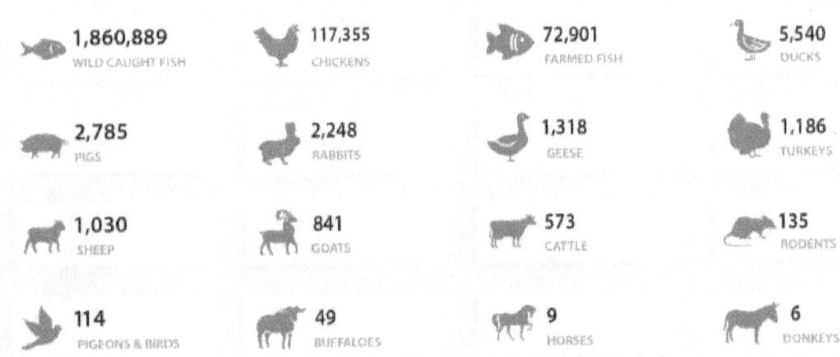

Courtesy: TheVeganCalculator.com and AnimalClock.org.

These numbers are enormous and mind boggling. But as individuals we can do something about it. Small drops make the ocean.

Same way, you and I can make a difference by going vegan and refusing to consume products that involve cruelty and killing animals. There is great awakening happening in the world right now and we can be part of this to save animals and our earth.

Animals slaughtered for food every year, day, and hour

Animal	Per Year	Per day	Per hour
Wild fish	2,664,500 million	7,300 million	304,166,667
Farmed fish	109,500 million	300 million	12,500,000
Chickens	65,000 million	178 million	7,416,667
Ducks	4,000 million	11 million	458,333
Pigs	1,460 million	4 million	166,667
Rabbits	1,100 million	3 million	125,000
Geese	730 million	2 million	83,333
Turkeys	730 million	2 million	83,333
Sheep	550 million	1.5 million	62,500
Goats	440 million	1.2 million	50,000
Cows	300 million	0.8 million	33,333
Total	2,850,000 mil.	7,800 mil.	325,145,833

Worldwide, each year, 70 billion land animals and 3 trillion marine animals are killed.

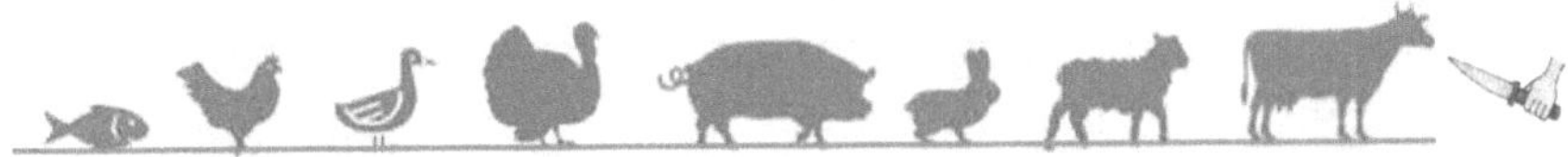

CHAPTER 8

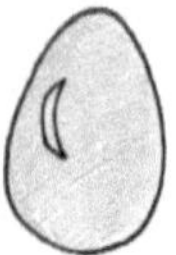

EGGS ARE CRUEL. PERIOD.

Milk and eggs are similar in many ways. If milk is exploitation of female reproductive system of cows, then eggs are exploitation of female reproductive system of hens.

Egg-laying hens are the most abused animals in the world.

In factory farms, hens usually receive less than one square foot (around 750 sq. cm) of space, much less than the size of the in-flight tray tables.

They spend every hour of every day standing in cramped, uncomfortable sheds, living in feces and urine. Imagine someone standing above you excreting and urinating all the time. It is a pathetic condition.

In addition, the lights in poultry farms are often altered in order to manipulate the chickens into laying eggs more frequently. Antibiotics are often mixed with the feed itself, because you cannot figure out which hens have some disease. The hens have portions of their beaks cut off with hot blades while they're fully conscious to prevent them from pecking each other in their overcrowded environments.

The natural lifespan of a chicken is 10 to 15 years. But poultry farms retire their hens to the slaughterhouse in 18 months. So, the hens are barely teenagers when they are killed, after growing them at a humongous rate of 400% every day! They're killed, soaked in a chlorine bath to remove odor of feces and urine, and the corpses are shipped to the grocery store, destined for your dinner plate, packed nicely and labeled attractively.

There are two kinds of chickens. One is "broilers" used for meat and "layers" used for laying eggs, each with distinct "engineered" genetics, metabolism, and functions.

The male offspring of layers are not "designed for meat" and they cannot lay eggs as well. So what happens to male chicks, which are half of the population of layers? Simple, they are destroyed! In some farms, male layer chickens are sucked through series of pipes to land them in electrified plates. In some farms, chicks are tossed into large plastic containers, where they are suffocated and killed, as they cry out for their lost mothers on the Day 1 of their life. In some farms they are ground alive in machines and used as feed for other animals.

Eggs are not healthy for humans. People who regularly consume eggs are twice as likely to develop type 2 diabetes. Eggs contain saturated fat and cholesterol, both of which are linked to heart disease. A single large egg yoke contains approximately 250 mg of cholesterol and that is more than a days' need and eating so much of cholesterol regularly contributes to heart and other diseases. Eggs can induce hormone-sensitive cancers as well.

Like female humans, hens also menstruate and have their periods. Eggs are what come out during these "periods." Why eat "Chicken periods," asks Gary Yourofsky. He further says things that come out of a hen's cloaca, the singular hole of a bird's backside that serves as the poophole, peehole and egghole, are not sane breakfast choices. Consuming an object that fell out of another species' excretory hole is at the best disgusting.

CHAPTER 9

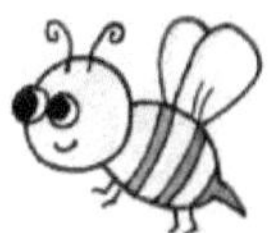

WHAT ABOUT HONEY, DEAR?!

Bees started making honey around 200 million years ago, long before humans even appeared on planet Earth. Anatomically modern humans, *Homo sapiens*, came into existence only 1 million years ago.

It takes a bee it's entire lifetime to produce just one spoonful of honey. A single honeybee visits around 7,000 flowers a day.

To produce just 100 grams of honey, it takes 4 lakhs flower visits and a total of 20,000 km of flying by bees. That is real hard work, right?

Honey is the only energy source of bees. Bees store honey and consume it over the winter months, when honey production comes down. Honey is the bank balance and fixed deposits of honeybees.

Honey that we get is the result of exploitation of bees, and there is no difference between bee farming and other forms of animal farming. When we take honey, we steal the hard work and hard earned bank balance of bees.

In addition, commercial bee farmers employ practices that are unethical and inhumane. These include clipping the wings of queen bees to prevent them from fleeing the hive and killing entire colonies to prevent the spread of diseases. Oftentimes bees are killed or have their wings and legs torn off by haphazard handling.

When honey is taken away from bees, it is often replaced by sugar or high-fructose corn syrup (HFCS) to prevent the bees from starving during the colder months. Sugar is also given to bees in the spring to encourage colony growth. These sugars don not provide bees the many beneficial nutrients found in flower nectar.

Even worse, these sweeteners and sugar harm the bees' immune systems and can cause genetic changes. They reduce their defenses against pesticides.

Such commercial honey farming harms the health of bees and their long-term sustainability. Do you think honey produced by such means will be good for human consumption? It will only spoil our health in the long run.

It is not right and not ethical to steal the honey, which is the result of long hard work of bees.

* * *

If you are vegan, caring for insects and their well-being, you do not harm honeybees and you do not consume honey.

Date syrup and maple syrup, which are plant-based, are good alternatives for honey.

Let us also stop using products containing beeswax, which include lip balms and other cosmetics.

Honey may be sweet, but remember it comes from bee's stomach and hence it is actually bee vomit. Is it not disgusting to consume vomit? Unlike bees, humans can survive and thrive without honey in their diets.

CHAPTER 10

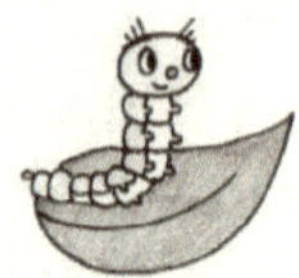

SILK IS NOT SANE AND LEATHER IS LAME

Imagine resting and awaiting a magnificent metamorphosis, only to be violently boiled alive so that humans get silk to wear. Cruel isn't it?

While it is very clear to many people why vegans don't eat meat or dairy, why they do not wear silk or use leather are not very obvious.

Not everyone knows silk and leather are animal products and they are a result of intense cruelty shown to animals.

Silk is used in making great looking silk sarees, silk dhotis and other fabrics and such silk is made from the fiber that is spun by silkworms or mulberry worms. Silkworms make their cocoons during their pupal stage prior to becoming moths or butterflies.

In order to harvest silk, silkworms are killed. Their cocoons or homes are immersed in boiling water, which kill the silkworms. Since vegans do not use products that exploit animals, they do not use silk.

More than 10,000 silkworms are killed to make a silk saree. Around 3 trillion (3,000,000,000,000) worms are killed, world over, for silk in a year. "Cruelty is one fashion statement we can all do without" said Rue McClanahan, an American actress.

Silkworms may look different from humans, but, just like us, they have central nervous systems and brains. They are living beings, and they also want to live.

"Silk is more horrible than meat. By using silk you are accumulating even more sin than eating meat. For meat few animals are killed, whereas for silk thousands of silkworms are killed", said Kanchi Acharya Sri Chandrasekara Saraswathi.

"The victim feels the suffering in his own mind and body, whereas the victimizer can be quite unaware of that suffering. The sword does not feel the pain that it inflicts" said Philip Hallie, author and philosopher.

Even the harvesting of Eri silk or Ahimsa silk is not acceptable since it involves the domestication, breeding, and exploitation of animals.

Many famous online fashion retailers and brick and mortar shops are doing away with silk in United Kingdom and United States.

Leather is another form of less obvious cruelty to animals. More than a billion cows, pigs, goats, sheep, alligators, ostriches, kangaroos, and even dogs and cats are cruelly slaughtered for their skin every year.

Turning skin into leather takes loads of energy and gives away a toxic mix of chemicals. Tannery waste contains water-fouling salt, lime sludge, sulfides, acids, and other pollutants.

Alternatives to leather such as synthetic, vegan or faux leather are available. Eco-friendly alternatives, such as jute are great, as well as, are less expensive.

CHAPTER 11

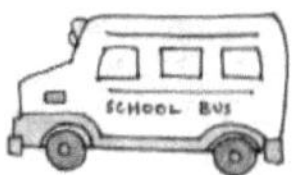

SCHOOL TRIP TO A SLAUGHTERHOUSE?!

You must have heard about school trips to parks, museums, or industries. Have you ever heard about a school trip to a slaughterhouse?

You would not. Because if we take school children to a slaughterhouse, they will be shocked and, seeing the horror first hand, they will give up eating animals right away.

If children give up eating meat, it will impact meat industry at large and they will never allow this.

If you leave an apple and a rabbit with a toddler or baby, which one will she eat and which one will she play with? Obviously, the baby will eat the apple and play with the rabbit and never the other way around. Eating meat is not natural and not in the genes or instinct of babies and children.

A good number of children start eating meat because of the insistence of their parents. Children are force-fed meat at a young age.

Children do not even know meat is produced by killing animals. In a survey done in the United States, when children were asked, "Do you eat animals?" the majority said "no" and they were also shocked at the concept of eating animals.

Meat is produced in faraway places, out of sight so that no one ever knows how animals are killed and murdered and how meat is produced.

Paul McCartney, an English singer and musician, famously said, "If all slaughterhouses had glass walls, everybody would be vegetarian."

Though movies with violence or murder are shown regularly on TVs, how meat is produced in slaughterhouses is never shown on TVs or in the movies. If they show, most of us will stop eating meat. No one can go to a slaughterhouse and take videos of animals being killed and how meat is produced. Such animal breeding sites and slaughterhouses are kept as secret as NASA or a Pentagon Defence facility!

If how our food is produced cannot be shown live on a TV, it means there is something seriously wrong about it.

In a way, we are indifferent and uncaring about how meat is produced. We do not want to see and we do not want our children to see the pain the animals undergo in slaughterhouses during their murder.

There is a comfort in ignorance, especially when it comes to how the food we eat is produced.

According to philosopher Élisabeth de Fontenay, we are not bloodthirsty or sadistic. We are simply indifferent, passive, aloof, uncaring, unkind, callous, thick-skinned, complicit, bloated, sleepy, and unconscious about animals' right to life.

But this has to change. You should be comfortable taking your children to places where our food is produced.

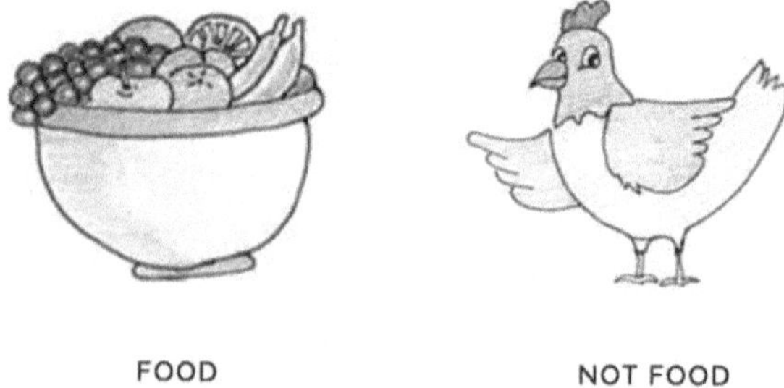

If you had to show your child where his or her food came from, where are you more likely to take them, a farm where fruits and vegetables are harvested or a slaughterhouse?

CHAPTER 12

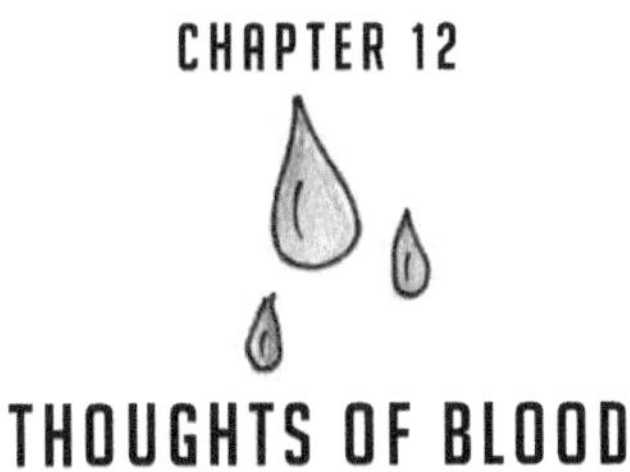

THOUGHTS OF BLOOD

When I was writing this book, flood of thoughts, sorry thoughts of blood crossed me. I was brought up and grew up next to a cow slaughterhouse in a small town in Tamil Nadu bordering Kerala in India.

I used to cross the cow slaughterhouse few times every day. I used to jump over small blood streams that were constantly flowing and take a small detour over heaps of smelling cow dung. I used to close my nose tight because of the bad smell. Even today I can recall the strong odor from the slaughterhouse.

Whenever I cross the place, usually to buy groceries for my mom or to play with friends, I used to peep into the slaughter house. I would see a cow and her legs would be tied with ropes to a pillar. Head or neck would also be tied to the roof or a rod above her. Soon, a man would slit the throat of the cow and leave it for a while, and in the meantime would get the next one ready for slaughter. The blood would start flowing and the cow would die in pain and tears. Also, the cow would cry, mourn, and make loud noises, at times.

After getting groceries, when I cross again, I will be seeing the same cow but all skin removed with her meat and interior fully exposed.

Sometimes, I see a baby cow alive. I think when they rip open a mother cow, there would be a live baby inside. Not sure what they did with such small babies but it is easy to guess as the place is a slaughterhouse.

As a kid, I did not know what was going on. On one hand I knew something was wrong, but on the other hand I thought whatever grown-up adults do must be right. I have crossed this place and jumped over the blood streams hundreds of times with those mixed feelings and thoughts.

Then, every evening, they used to load a truck with cow meat, packing it with ice and send them to the neighboring state of Kerala.

Recently I asked my dad, with a bit of anger, what as adults, they were doing those days watching these scenes in the slaughter house. As a grown-up now, I think I am as helpless as he was then. The slaughterhouses are not any more next to our homes. They are now located far away, concealed in sophistication. But videos of scenes of what I saw are all over on YouTube and social media now.

Same processes with variations are followed for goat, pig, and chickens. If you see this process with your own eyes in real time, for few days, you will stop eating food, forget eating animals. Do we need to inflict so much cruelty and pain just to satisfy two inches of our tongue and to fill six inches of our stomachs?

Leo Tolstoy, the famous Russian writer and philosopher, said, "As long as there are slaughterhouses, there will be battlefields." If you ask any child, he or she will be against killing animals for food.

CHAPTER 13

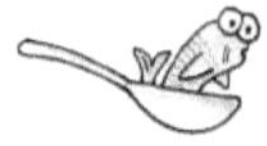

I WON'T EAT ANIMALS…

In an interesting and thought-provoking video, which has 1.2 million views on YouTube, Zada a five-year-old girl realizes meat is made from animals.

Here is her conversation with her mother:

Zada : I won't eat animals.

Mother : What would you eat instead?

Zada : I will eat whatever there is on the table but not chicken or meat.

Mother : Why do you think you do not want to do that?

Zada : Because they are animals and I like animals.

Mother : So what will you or we do if we miss eating chicken or meat?

Zada : I don't miss chicken and meat.

Mother : How about fish?

Zada : Fish? Is it an animal?

Mother : Yeah.

Zada : I won't eat that either.

Mother : Oh, my god

Zada : I won't eat animals. (Stubbornly)

Mother : Ok. What do you want to eat? What kind of food do you want to eat?

Zada : Any thing on the table, but not animals.

Mother : Why do you feel sorry for the animals?

Zada : Because they are nice and I know that we cook them some times which is not very nice. And I know we like to eat animals that we cook, but that is not nice for them.

Mother : Do you think they suffer?

Zada : I think they don't really like being cooked in the oven.

To watch this video, search for Zada + 'I won't eat animals' on YouTube.

* * *

In another interesting video titled "Why He Doesn't Want to Eat Octopus", Luiz Antonio, a small boy, tells why he does not want to eat octopus. The video makes an interesting watch and has 75K+ views.

These videos provide evidence that children love animals and they do not like to eat animals. Watch these videos of Zada and Luiz with your children and check what their views are on eating animals.

CHAPTER 14

WHAT IS TRUE "HALAL"?

Generally, Muslims are not often associated with veganism. But this is changing.

Islam teaches kindness, which extends to all living creatures. If you read the Qur'an, it says animals are sentient, that is, emotional beings just as human beings are. Prophet Muhammed himself was not an advocate of daily meat consumption. He never insisted on having a specific type of food; he ate whatever he was provided.

Umar ibn Al-Khattab, a companion of Prophet Muhammed, explicitly warned against eating meat, calling it addictive (al-Muwaṭṭa' 1742).

Historically, Muslims ate almost no meat or very less meat. The wealthy had meat once a week, and the poor only consumed on Eids. The Prophet's diet primarily consisted of dates, barley, and water.

What about halal? Halal is an Arabic word that means "permissible" or "considered good."

Most of today's meat, even when labeled "halal," comes from farms where the animals endure cramped conditions, cruel and inhumane practices, and are injected with harmful steroids and hormones.

Slaughter, production, and sale of meat are cruel and disgusting. Many take solace in the idea that they can purchase halal meat, dismissing the brutal, overcrowded, inhumane conditions that the animals are raised and slaughtered in. This definitely is not halal.

The Qur'an places emphasis on the environment and how we should care for it. If raising animals for human consumption is a major cause of global warming, then as per Qur'an, animal agriculture is not good, not permissible, not halal, and should not be pursued.

Animals are mentioned in the Qur'an in relation to sacrifice, only because in that time, place, and circumstances, animals were the means of survival. In those desert lands, humans were intricately tied up in the natural cycle, and as a part of that, they killed and were killed like every other species of that area.

"In fact, there are well-known devout Muslims who practice vegetarianism. Hazrat Ali Ibn Abi Talib, the cousin and son-in-law of Prophet Muhammad, the fourth Khalifa as per Sunni belief, has been quoted in *Sharh Nahjul Balagha,* as saying: 'Do not make your stomach a graveyard of animals,' " quoted *Daily Pioneer.*

After seeing the atrocities done to animals in the meat industry, many Muslims are turning Vegan in the United Kingdom, France, Australia, Canada, and other countries.

"...Eat and drink from the provision of Allah, and do not commit abuse on the earth, spreading corruption" – Quran 2:60

https://www.Animals*in*Islam.com/ has some great materials for a follow-up reading.

CHAPTER 15

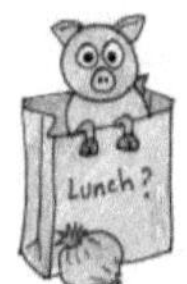

WHAT DID YOU EAT FOR LUNCH?

Rabi'a al Adawiyya is one of the most famous female saints in Islam. She was born in 717 CE, just 80 years after the death of the Prophet. During her childhood, her parents died, and she was sold into slavery.

After her release from slavery, Rabi'a went to the desert for prayer and meditation. Rabi'a was a Sufi, a member of a sect that preaches total love of God and total union with Him.

Later, she returned to Basra, leading a life of voluntary poverty and simplicity. Her life was marked by acts of kindness toward humans and animals alike.

When she was in the mountains, the animals gathered around her: deer, gazelles, mountain goats, and wild donkeys. In her presence, they were trusting and fearless.

Once, when Hasan-Al-Basri, another Sufi teacher, approached her, the animals ran away. He asked her why the animals gathered around her but ran away when he came.

Rabi'a responded by asking him what he ate for lunch. "Pig fat and onions," he replied.

"You eat their fat! Why should they not run away from you?" exclaimed Rabi'a.

In addition to Rabi'a al Adawiyya, many other saints in Islam, including Rumi, were vegetarians.

Rumi asked, "How can I kill even the tiniest creature, just to satisfy my tongue?" Even a seemingly lifeless stone has a degree of consciousness; respect it. He even refrained from sacrificing animals on Eid-Al-Adah (Bakrid).

Rumi writes that what we eat directly influences our thinking. If we consume an animal, its blood and meat will make us act like a slaughterer or killer.

* * *

$$a^2+b^2=c^2$$

Remember this math theorem? Yes! It is the Pythagoras theorem for a right-angled triangle.

But did you know a fact about Pythagoras?

Pythagoras was not only vegetarian, but he also refused to wear clothing of leather and wool. He abstained from eating meat and from involving in sacrifice that costs life of an animal being.

Pythagoras proclaimed, "Blood offerings could not possibly give pleasure to God, who is supposed to be full of kindness."

People like Rabi'a al Adawiyya and Pythagoras were mature enough to respect animals' right to life and hence did not consume meat and any other animal products.

CHAPTER 16

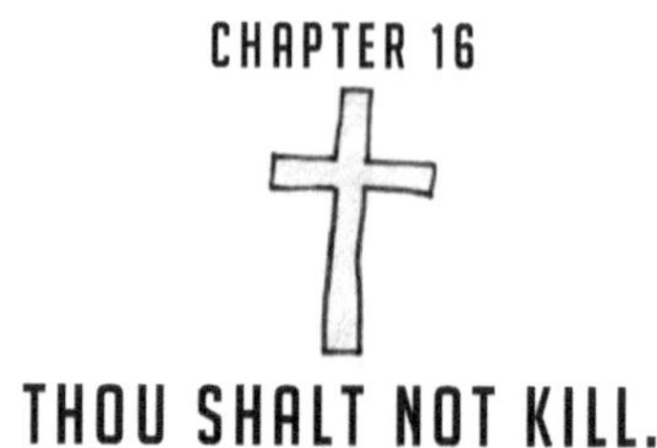

THOU SHALT NOT KILL.

Regardless of ones' opinions about religion, most will agree that unnecessary killing is wrong. To Christians, killing is deemed a sin and thus listed among the Ten Commandments – "THOU SHALT NOT KILL."

God did not say this commandment need to be practiced only with humans. Why did we assume that this commandment does not apply to animals?

Animals are at the same level as humans. In Ecclesiastes, God proclaims, "For people and animals share the same fate – both breathe and both must die. So people have no real advantage over the animals" (3:19). He continues, "For who can prove that the human spirit goes up and the spirit of animals goes down into the earth?" (3:21).

In Genesis 1:29, God tells exactly what to eat right after He created man : "Behold, I have given you every plant yielding seed that is on the surface of all the earth, and every tree which has fruit yielding seed; it shall be food for you." Adam and Eve lived in a garden full of vegetables and fruits and were living on a plant-based diet. Then sin arrives in the form of a Satan and mention of meat comes only after Satan arrives.

Christians are inspired by long religious traditions of fasting from meat and other animal products. Many Coptic Christians today observe fasts imposing a vegan diet for two-thirds of the year. The practice of not eating animal products redirects one's focus away from selfish pleasure and toward God.

Such traditions remind Christians that animals belong to God, so humans must treat them with respect and cannot do whatever they want.

"Do not, for the sake of food, destroy the work of God. Everything is indeed clean, but it is wrong for anyone to make another stumble (blunder) by what he eats. It is good not to eat meat or drink wine or do anything that causes your brother to stumble" (Romans 14:20–21). As per St. Jerome's letter to Eustoquie, the use of flesh and wine has commenced after the Deluge.

"Not to hurt our humble brethren (animals) is our first duty to them, but to stop there is not enough. We have a higher mission – to be of service to them whenever they require it. If you have men who will exclude any of world's creatures and animals from the shelter of compassion and pity, you will have men who will deal likewise with their fellow men," said St. Fransis of Assisi (1181 – 1226) a well-known saint.

"But I do say to you; Kill neither men, nor beasts, nor yet the food which goes into your mouth. For if you eat living food, the same will quicken you, but if you kill your food, the dead food will kill you also. For life comes from life and from death comes always death. For everything which kills your bodies kills your souls also" says The Essene Gospel of Peace.

The Essene Gospel of Peace adds, "For I tell you truly, he who kills, kills himself; and whoso eats the flesh of slain beasts, eats of the body of death. For in his blood every drop of their blood turns to poison; in his breath their breath to stink; in his flesh their flesh to boils; in his bones their bones to chalk... And their death will become his death"

Concern for fellow humans, fellow animal creatures, and the environment are obligations for Christians, and hence being a Christian, it makes sense to refrain from killing animals for food and refrain from animal abuse.

The act of killing and feasting on dead animals does not sound like the work of a kind God and it is more like that of the Devil. A vision of delighting in God's world and living responsibly among the fellow creatures, by adopting a vegan way of life, will be an inspiration to all Christians.

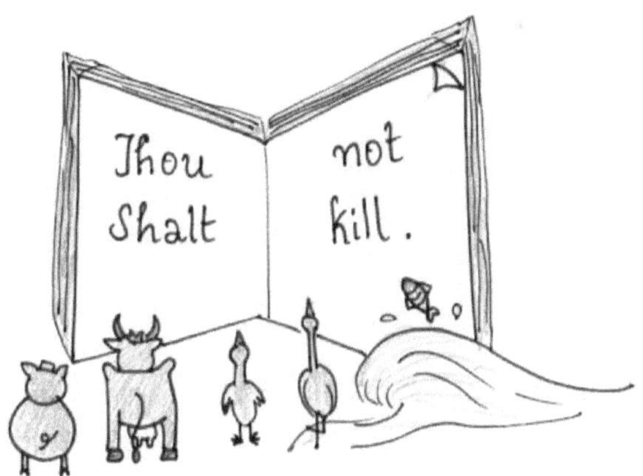

"Thou shalt not kill"! [...]

There is not an asterisk next
to that commandment saying:
"unless you walk on all four
and have fur, feathers, horns,
beaks or gills."

Gary Yourofsky

Thou shalt not kill.

CHAPTER 17

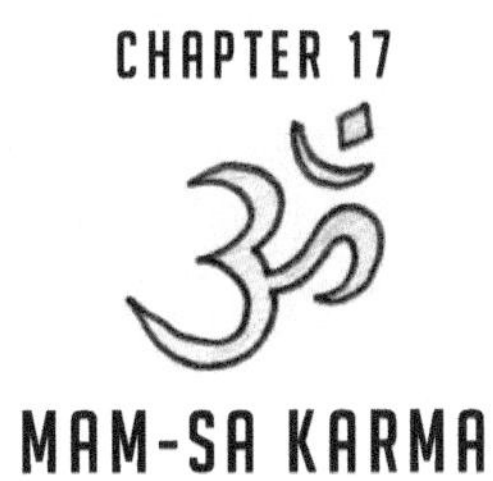

MAM-SA KARMA

Hinduism strongly recommends ahimsa – the concept of non-violence toward all life forms, including animals. Hindu religion promotes ahimsa way of living. *Mahabharata* has a popular proverb: "Nonviolence is the highest duty and the highest teaching." A vegan way of living is non-violent.

Hindu religion, in many places, highlights the ill effects of meat eating. *Manusmriti* says "There is no greater sinner than a man who wants to make his own flesh thrive at the expense of someone else's."

Many Hindu religious texts proclaim that non-vegetarian food is harmful for the body, the mind and spiritual development. Plant-based food, on the other hand, is considered satvic, good, and purifying to the body and mind.

One can never obtain meat without causing pain and injury to the animals. One should, therefore, abstain from meat. *Manu Samhita*, an ancient Hindu Dharamasastra, says, "He who permits the slaughter of an animal, he who kills it, he who cuts it up, he who buys or sells meat, he who cooks it, he who serves it up, and he who eats it, must all be considered as the killers or murderers of the animal..."

Mahabharata contains some of the strongest statements against the harming of animals and the consumption of their flesh. The *Mahabharata* in fact has three entire chapters dedicated to the evils of eating meat.

Hindus also believe in karma. As per law of karma, if you eat an animal, one must be killed by the same animal later. This is called mam-sa. Mam means me and sa means he. As I am eating an animal, that animal will have an opportunity to eat me.

"Jaisa ann, vaisa man (जैसा अन्न वैसा मन) – Food defines your thoughts. We all know animals have feelings and emotions. Close your eyes for thirty seconds and ask yourself what feelings animals go through in the slaughterhouse?" asks Sister Brahma Kumari Shivani Ji.

"Animals in the slaughterhouse go through the following emotions – hatred, anger, resentment, fear, hurt, pain, and helplessness for many days and finally violence and death. After all these, it comes on our plate and we say it is protein and health. This does not match," she concludes.

Some of you may want to say that people did eat meat during Vedic days or dairy is part of Hindu tradition. We should look at religion and its scriptures for broad aspects like love and compassion and not for day-to-day operational matters.

If you try to interpret what has been said thousands of years back by hundreds of people, without applying our mind, we will be travelling in the wrong direction and will be in for a trouble soon.

Vedas and scriptures did not talk about using cars or mobile phones. But still, we use them today! Similarly what is said or practiced thousands of years back, on operational issues, is not relevant for today. Take the broad lessons and apply it for today, tomorrow, and future.

CHAPTER 18

SACRIFICING ANIMAL SACRIFICE?

All religions call for compassion. No religion requires killing or eating animals. Hacking animals to death with weapons is just plain cruelty and murder.

Animal sacrifice is bad for everyone. It normalizes killing and desensitizes people and children toward violence against animals and even humans.

Children seeing animal sacrifice would think killing animals is right. All the more, it provokes violence in their minds. A child seeing killing of animals will think killing a human is also right. That is how violence in the society still continues.

Animal sacrifice occurs in all countries and in all religions.

During Nepal's Gadhimai festival alone, just in a couple of days, 300,000 animals are killed every year.

The Eid al-Adha is a major annual festival of animal sacrifice in Islam. Nearly 10,000,000 animals are sacrificed in Pakistan every year on Eid. In Indonesia, 1,000,000+ animals were sacrificed in 2019 for the festival. In Turkey, 2,500,000 sheep, cows and goats are sacrificed each year. Saudi Arabia transports nearly a

54

million animals every year for sacrifice to Mina (near Mecca). The sacrificed animals at Eid al-Adha include the four species considered lawful for the Hajj sacrifice: sheep, goats, camels, and cattle.

In India, in most of the Kali temples or Amman temples, animal sacrifices are common. In 2016, in Erode, a town in India, villagers sacrificed 3,000 goats to placate the rain gods.

In a ceremony which comes once in seven years at a Kaliamman temple in Kulakaranpatti village in Karur district of Tamil Nadu, 1,000 buffalos are sacrificed.

In February 2020, the Kuzhumayee Amman temple located in Trichy, India saw murder of 1,200 goats in the name of sacrifice. This festival named "Kutti Kudithal" meaning tasting the blood of lambs, involves the temple priest drinking the blood of hundreds of goats (alive) to appease the goddess. In another temple festival, at Poosariyur near Anthiyur (also in Tamil Nadu), at least 5,000 baby goats are slaughtered, every year.

Animal sacrifices are crude. Although, old, archaic, ancient religious texts had mentioned about animal sacrifices, the society has advanced. We are in a modern era and in 2020s. The rituals, which were prevalent in the early period of civilization, have lost their significance. We need to move on from these crude rituals, to new rituals that are based on reasoning, love, and kindness.

"We could destroy animals more easily than they could destroy us. That is the sole firm basis for our claim of superiority. There is no objective reason to believe that the interests of human being are more important than those of animals," says Bertrand Russell, a British philosopher and a Nobel laureate.

Over the centuries and millennia, we moved on from post cards to WhatsApp, bullock carts to bikes, rocks to robots, but why stay on with animal sacrifice? Let us also move from cruelty to compassion.

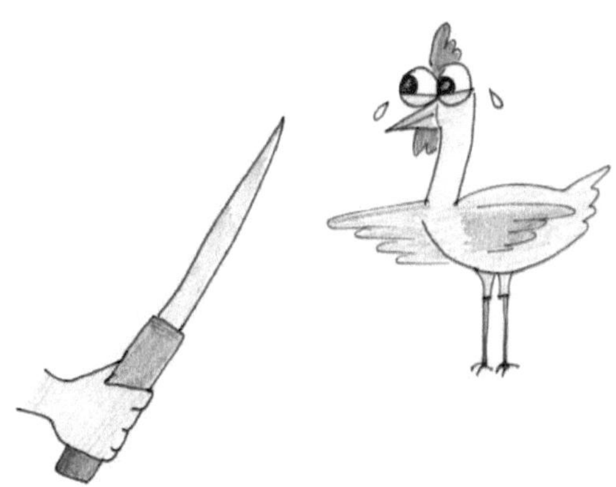

The question is not,
Can they reason?
Nor can they talk?

But can they suffer?

Jeremy Benthlam Philosopher 1789

CHAPTER 19

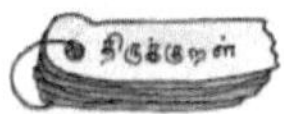

HOW WILL GOD'S GRACE COME TO YOU?

Thiruvalluvar, a Tamil poet, who lived almost two thousand years back in India, has explained in clear and unequivocal terms about ill effects of eating meat and how we need to treat animals.

தன்னூன் பெருக்கற்குத் தான்பிறிது ஊனுண்பான்
எங்ஙனம் ஆளும் அருள்.

தன் உடம்பைப் பெருக்கச் செய்வதற்காகத் தான்
மற்றோர் உயிரின் உடம்பைத் தின்கின்றவன் எவ்வாறு
அருளுடையவனாக இருக்க முடியும்?

If we eat flesh and corpse of other creatures to increase our own flesh, how will God's blessing come to us? How will God's grace come to you? Asks Thiruvalluvar.

Another verse of Thirukural explains how what we eat decides the composition of our mind.

படைகொண்டார் நெஞ்சம்போல் நன்னூக்காது ஒன்றன்
உடல்சுவை உண்டார் மனம்.

Like the murderous mind of him who carries a weapon in his hand, the mind of him who feasts with pleasure on the body of another (creature), has no regard for goodness and kindness.

No wonder, as the world is becoming more meat eating, the cruelty and violence are also equally increasing.

The above thoughts of Thiruvalluvar were also reflected later by well-known and renowned Christian saint St. Fransis of Assisi (1181 - 1226)

St. Fransis of Assisi proclaimed "If you have men who will exclude any of world's creatures and animals from the shelter of compassion and pity, you will have men who will deal likewise with their fellow men."

* * *

Many of us might say: "I am not killing animals. Because meat is being sold, I am buying and eating it. If it is not sold, I would not buy."

Thiruvallur has an answer even for this.

தினற்பொருட்டால் கொல்லாது உலகெனின் யாரும்
விலைப்பொருட்டால் ஊன்றருவா ரில்.

புலால் தின்னும் பொருட்டு உலகத்தார் உயிர்களைக்
கொல்லா திருப்பாரானால், விலையின் பொருட்டு ஊன்
விற்பவர் இல்லாமல் போவார்.

If there is no one eating flesh or meat, then no one would sell flesh to make money.

Chapter Pulaal Maruthal (abstinence from flesh or meat), verses 251 through 260 has more insights on why we need to give up eating meat.

CHAPTER 20

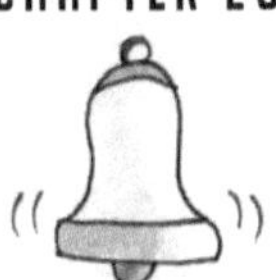

COW THAT RANG THE BELL

Manuneethi Cholan (205 BE), one of the famous Tamil kings, hung a huge bell in front of his palace. He announced that anyone seeking justice can ring the bell and he would deliver justice swiftly.

Once, his son, the young prince, went around the city in his chariot and he was speeding carelessly. Suddenly, a baby cow (a calf), which was crossing the street, came in the way and got crushed under the wheels of the prince's chariot. The mother of the calf helplessly watched her little one die.

The saddened cow immediately walked to the palace entrance and rang the bell demanding justice from the king.

The king came out and saw a cow ringing the bell. Surprised, he followed the cow and learnt about the death of the young calf under the wheels of his son's chariot.

To deliver justice to the cow in distress, the king ordered his son to be killed. But no one was ready to do this. Hence, the king himself took the chariot and killed his son, in the same way in which the calf had died. By this way, as he witnessed his son die, the king went through the same pain that the cow had gone through. Seeing this, God appeared and brought the son and calf back to life.

If a human needs justice, why not a cow or an animal? King Shibi was famous and known for his generous nature and justice. Once a pigeon flew into King Shibi's court and sat on his lap. He sensed that the pigeon was trembling with fear and lovingly held it in his hands.

Soon, an eagle flew toward King Shibi's court and asked the king to hand over the pigeon as it was its prey. But Shibi refused. He said that the pigeon has taken refuge with him and he will not hand over the pigeon to it. He also suggested the eagle to look for food, other than the pigeon's flesh.

The eagle was adamant and said that it wanted only the pigeon. King Shibi, seeing the plight of the pigeon, said he will give the eagle his own flesh. He took a knife quickly, cut the flesh from his thigh, used a weighing scale to make sure it weighed same as the pigeon's weight and gave it to the eagle.

Indian kings set examples of love and non-violence toward humans as well as animals.

King Ashoka (260 BE) established some of the first animal rights laws. He stopped royal hunting and ended killing of animals for the royal kitchen and abstained from eating meat.

His famous pillar edict declares: "I have enforced the law against killing animals. The greatest progress of righteousness among men comes from the exhortation in favour of non-injury to life and abstention from killing living beings."

Ashoka insisted his people to be compassionate toward animals and to refrain from killing them.

CHAPTER 21

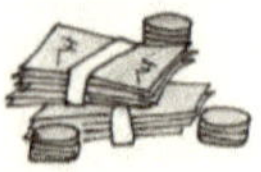

STOP PAYING FOR ANIMAL ABUSE, NOW

All of us are compassionate, kind, and in general against animal abuse. We are great souls.

But our life style is such that we are getting disconnected and we are becoming ignorant about what we do.

During our day-to-day life, we do not harm or kill animals directly. But indirectly we are causing a great deal of disturbance to animals, to our earth, and hence to all fellow human beings.

Meat, egg, cheese, or milk is available readily in the supermarket, nicely packed like a pack of bread or a bottle of water; we buy them and go on consuming. We go to restaurants and enjoy meat or dairy without knowing or bothering about the behind-the-scene pains, cruelty, or problems.

Did you know that every time you order that plate of biriyani, drink that cup of coffee, or eat that bowl of ice cream or slice of pizza, you are quite literally paying some one to slit the throat of a chicken or a goat or torture cows – something you yourself never want to do to those animals.

The meat and dairy industries are doing an intelligent job of concealing the pain, torture, and murder of animals and show pictures of happy cows in a green grass field or a smiling chicken on top of the food packaging.

Our text books or schools talk about Jallianwala Bagh massacre or other social unrests where hundreds of people have died. But they keep quiet and maintain a still silence about billions of animals being killed every year in slaughterhouses.

Neither politicians nor courts pay attention to animal abuse, because legally we can kill animals. The laws were made by us in ignorance and without considering the feelings of the victims, that is, animals. We humans have created a legal system where we gave power to ourselves to kill animals just because they look different, cannot speak, or have a tail or feathers.

"As consumers we have so much power to change the world by just being careful in what we buy," said Emma Watson, an actress and an activist.

It is easy to be ignorant. It is easy to just go on with life — blame it on or rationalize using age-old food habits or quote old, archaic, irrelevant-for-today religious texts and go on with life as usual. It is easy and convenient to pick up what is available in the super market aisles. It is tasty to order that biriyani or cheese pizza or ice-cream.

"Most of us are fond of animals. But our compassion stops at the edge of our plates," says Matthieu Ricard.

It is important not to contribute to the unnecessary and unjust suffering of animals by choosing plant-based food over meat, dairy, and other products sourced from animals. It is definitely easier to switch to plant-based options than being caged, tortured, and killed.

CHAPTER 22

BUT, YOU KNOW…?

"Human beings were originally meat eaters and hunters."

- Human civilization is about growing and evolving and not blindly sticking to the past.
- The behaviors of primitive humans were justified given their primitive way of life.
- Human beings originally used stones as tools and never used computers. Why don't we stick to the original way of living?
- Our ancestors did not wear clothes, used other humans as slaves, went in bullock carts, and never used mobile phones. Why selectively copy paste from early humans?
- Even if our ancestors ate meat, it is illogical to justify given the current conditions, food security, and climate change issues.
- Human beings were sometimes cannibals as well, that is, eating each other – why did we stop now?

"Humans need to eat meat and dairy to maintain good health."

- Plant-based food contains all the required nutrients such as protein, carbohydrates, fats, vitamins, and amino acids.

- People eating vegan food are excelling in sports, running ultra-marathons and climbing the Mount Everest.
- A robust body of medical research has concluded that consumption of animal flesh and secretions is harmful to us.
- Medical research clearly proves that eating meat and dairy is a major cause for cancer and cardiovascular diseases.
- You might very well remember your doctor asking you to stop eating meat and non-vegetarian food to cure or prevent diabetes, blood pressure, heart issues, and kidney stones.
- There are roughly 75 million vegans in the world and they are in better health than meat eaters or dairy consumers.

"Animals do not suffer the way we do."

- People, as recently as 1950s, thought new born children felt no pain and they were operated on without anesthesia.
- "We have seen that the senses and intuitions, various emotions and faculties, such as love, memory, attention, curiosity, imitation, reason, etc. of which man boasts, can be found in an incipient or even in a well-developed condition in the lower animals," said Darwin.
- "Answer me: Did nature arrange all the apparatus of sensation in animals in order that they should feel nothing?" – asked the famous French writer and philosopher Voltaire.
- Even in earthworms we do find substances (endorphins) associated with the process of pain.

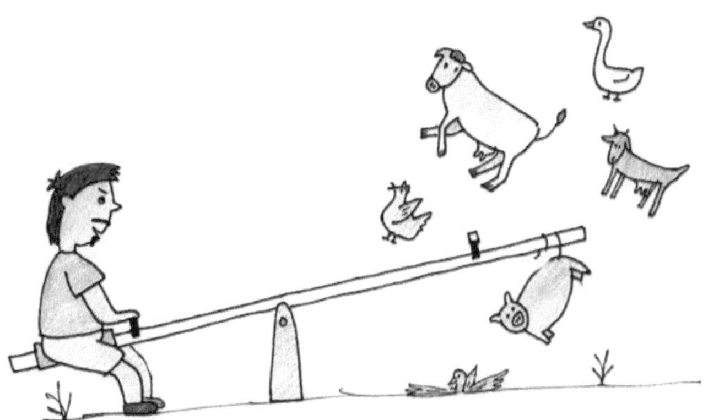

"What we are suggesting
here is not concern for
animals only but concern
for animals also."

Matthieu Ricard

But, you know…?

CHAPTER 23

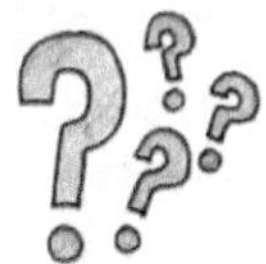

NEED MORE EXCUSES? HERE YOU GO.

"We can exploit animals as we are more intelligent than them."

- Can we exploit people with mental disabilities saying we are more intelligent or better than them?
- The capacity to suffer should be the measure and not how intelligent one is.
- Giving consideration and respect to animals is not an insult to human race. Being compassionate does not mean we are weak.
- Unlike plants, fungi, or microbes, animals are sentient beings, that is, they can feel pain.
- Exploiting animals does not even prove we are more powerful; Corona virus is a case in point.

"We are thinking about animals and ignoring people in poverty and misery. What about people suffering in Syria and Sudan? Should not we be concerned about people?"

- Being a vegan and helping animals in no way conflicts with helping people.
- By helping animals and not interfering in their lives, we help humans immensely by way of reduced climate change and better health.
- Because we care for our aged father, does not mean we should not take care of our mother who needs

> help or take care of a child who needs care. It is not "this or that"; it is "this and that."

- Human suffering does not and should not make animal suffering insignificant.
- Animal suffering is something that we are causing. Stopping this would not be of hindrance to helping humans in need.

"If we stop consuming dairy or eating meat, many businesses will be closed and thousands of jobs will be lost."

- People will always find alternate employment. We stopped using bicycles and where did the bicycle mechanics go?
- Legitimacy of an activity should not be judged by the jobs it creates or profits a business makes – Matthieu Ricard in 'A Plea for Animals'.
- Even slavery was once a profitable industry and employed thousands of people.
- Drug trafficking, theft, and paid killing also provide thousands of jobs and hence should we allow them?
- Should all of us use cigarettes or consume alcohol because it can provide job opportunities for many?
- "Should we employ bulldozers to demolish our own homes, schools and hospitals because 'if we don't do this, bulldozer operators will be out of job,' " asks Matthieu Ricard.
- In United States, for example, there are fewer American farmers today than two hundred years ago, despite America's population being nearly ten times more.
- Moving toward plant-based foods and sustainable farming practices will create more jobs than it would end.

"There are only two options: Make progress or make excuses."

CHAPTER 24

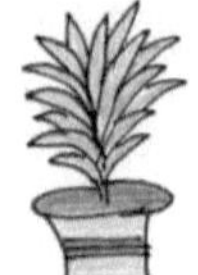

DON'T PLANTS ALSO HAVE LIFE?

You are right. Plants have life. Plants can feel sensations.

But they are not as evolutionarily developed as human animals or non-human animals. Plants do not have a central nervous system and a brain like human animals or non-human animals do. Since they do not have central nervous system and a brain, they cannot feel pain. They are not sentient.

If plants had a central nervous system and a brain, then they will fight back or run away from harvesting men or machines, like animals trying to escape when they know you are going to kill them.

Pain is a defense mechanism. If something hurts humans or animals, we react immediately – as "fight or flight."

Plants by nature are rooted, that is, they cannot move from one place to another because there is no need for it. Nature would not arrange things in such a way that you feel pain but you cannot move, run, or fly away to avoid pain.

If you try to kill an animal, either it will fight with you or it will try to run away. Plants by design do not feel pain and hence nature did not provide them with capabilities to "fight or flight."

* * *

All of us have to eat for survival. Which is better – to eat plants or animals? Feeding plants to animals and then eating animals is a very inefficient process.

Feeding massive amounts of grain and water to animals and then killing them, processing, transporting, and storing their flesh is not environmentally friendly. It consumes huge amount of resources of earth.

Eating plants directly is very efficient and results in less land usage, less water consumption, reduced carbon foot print, reduced climate change, and more importantly no pain for animals.

If you use 3 acres of land, you can feed 1 meat-eater for one year or 9 vegetarians (who consume dairy) for one year; whereas using the same area, we can feed 48 vegans, for one year. So land and water utilization is 16 times better if we embrace plant-based food.

Even if you are concerned about "plants having life" and "plants feel pain," by being a vegan we kill far less plants than we would by being a non-vegan. Entire forests, millions of trees, which "have life" and "can feel pain" are cut down in order to grow crops for animals so that we can eat them.

For our survival, we can eat plants, which will suffer less, rather than animals, which suffer more and equal to humans.

"Nothing will benefit human health and increase the chances for survival of life on earth as much as the evolution to a plant-based diet," said Albert Einstein.

CHAPTER 25

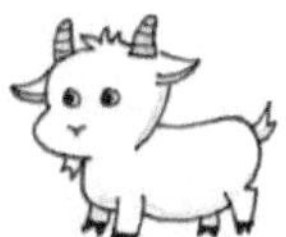

WITH MY MUM BY MY SIDE

A kid of a goat has a story for you:

I am walking on the road side,
With my mum by my side
Occasionally drinking her milk
And rubbing my nose on her fleece
*that's as smooth as silk**
Appears from nowhere a man so fat
With mustache like whiskers of a cat
With hands that look like they were
made from rubber and gum
He comes to my mum
By the leg he grabs her
And down the road he drags her
Paralyzed with shock, blind with tears
And heart full of odd fears
The fat man I follow,
As he drags my mum across a meadow
Then at a distance, I see a meat shop
That my mum had warned me to keep out of
The fat man ties my mum to a rod
I close my eyes and pray to God
The fat man unties my mum from the rod
I close my eyes and thank God
For a second, I think my mum is free
But the man takes her to a nearby tree

Before my eyes, he slays her head
   On my face, splashes her blood
He then rips my mum's flesh apart
   Here I stand with a broken heart
Then comes a man, thin and tall
   He trips on me and is about to fall
The thin man takes out some money and
   Places it on the fat man's hand
The fat man takes my mum's flesh down
   All I can do is cry and frown
The thin man takes my mum's flesh
   And speeds away in a rush
Though the street light is dim
   I try to run after him
But discover that it's of no use
   That it's of no use
These cruel humans cannot understand my plight
   Unless their loved ones are
Beheaded before their sight

I was walking on the road side,
   With my mum by my side
Occasionally drinking her milk
   And rubbing my nose on her fleece
   *that was as smooth as silk**

This poem is written by Manasa, an author and an animal rights activist, to portray the fact that animals live and care for each other as much as we, humans, do.

** The silk mentioned here is non-animal and cruelty-free silk.*

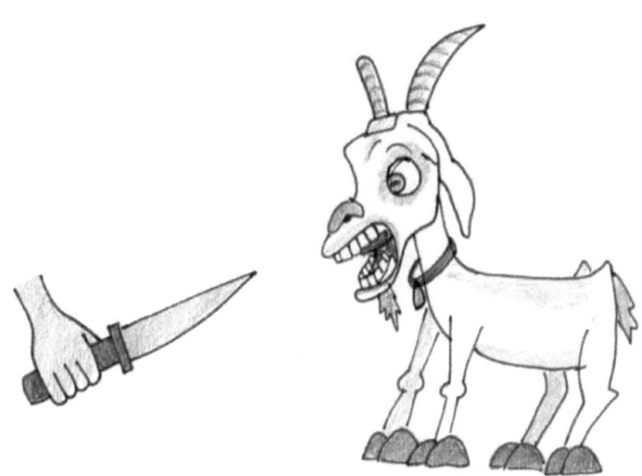

It is easy to choose meat
when you are not the one
with a knife at your throat.

With my mum by my side

Animals are my friends. And I don't eat my friends. Animals are my friends. And I don't eat my friends. Animals are my friends. And I don't eat my friends. Animals are my friends. And I don't eat my friends. Animals are my friends. And I don't eat my friends .Animals are my friends. And I don't eat my friends. Animals are my friends. And I don't eat my friends. Animals are my friends. And I don't eat my friends. Animals are my friends. And I don't eat my friends. Animals are my friends. And I don't eat my friends. Animals are my friends. And I don't eat my friends .Animals are my friends. And I don't eat my friends. Animals are my friends. And I don't eat my friends. Animals are my friends. And I don't eat my friends. Animals are my friends. And I don't eat my friends. Animals are my friends. And I don't eat my friends. Animals are my friends. And I don't eat my friends .Animals are my friends. And I don't eat my friends. Animals are my friends. And I don't eat my friends. Animals are my friends. And I don't eat my friends. Animals are my friends. And I don't eat my friends. Animals are my friends. And I don't eat my friends. Animals are my friends. And I don't eat my friends .Animals are my friends. And I don't eat my friends. Animals are my friends. And I don't eat my friends. Animals are my friends. And I don't eat my friends. Animals are my friends. And I don't eat my friends. Animals are my friends. And I don't eat my friends. Animals are my friends. And I don't eat my friends .Animals are my friends. And I don't eat my friends. Animals are my friends. And I don't eat my friends. Animals are my friends. And I don't eat my friends. Animals are my friends. And I don't eat my friends. Animals are my friends. And I don't eat my friends. Animals are my friends. And I don't eat my friends .Animals are my friends. And I don't eat my friends. Animals are my friends. And I don't eat my friends. Animals are my friends. And I don't eat my friends. Animals are my friends. And I don't eat my friends. Animals are my friends. And I don't eat my friends. Animals are my friends. And I don't eat my friends .Animals are my friends. And I don't eat my friends. Animals are my friends. And I don't eat my friends. Animals are my friends. And I don't eat my friends. Animals are my friends. And I don't eat my friends. Animals are my friends. And I don't eat my friends. Animals are my friends. And I don't eat my friends. *Animals are my friends. And I don't eat my friends. Animals are my friends. And I don't eat my friends. Animals are my friends. And I don't eat my friends. Animals are my friends. And I don't eat my friends. Animals are my friends. And I don't eat my friends. Animals are my friends. And I don't eat my friends .Animals are my friends. And I don't eat my friends. Animals are my friends. And I don't eat my friends. Animals are my friends. And I don't eat my friends. Animals are my friends. And I don't eat my friends. Animals are my friends. And I don't eat my friends. Animals are my friends. And I don't eat my friends .Animals are my friends. And I don't eat my friends. Animals are my friends. And I don't eat my friends. Animals are my friends. And I don't eat my friends. Animals are my friends. And I don't eat my friends. Animals are my friends. And I don't eat my friends. Animals are my friends. And I don't eat my friends. Animals are my friends. And I don't eat my friends .Animals are my friends. And I don't eat my friends. Animals are my friends. And I don't eat my friends. Animals are my friends. And I don't eat my friends. Animals are my friends. And I don't eat my friends. Animals are my friends. And I don't eat my friends .Animals are my friends. And I don't eat my friends. Animals are my friends. And I don't eat my friends. Animals are my friends. And I don't eat my friends. Animals are my friends. And I don't eat my friends. Animals are my friends. And I don't eat my friends. Animals are my friends. And I don't eat my friends. Animals are my friends. And I don't eat my friends. Animals are my friends. And I don't eat my friends. Animals are my friends. And I don't eat my friends. Animals are my friends. And I don't eat my friends. Animals are my friends. And I don't eat my friends. Animals are my friends. And I don't eat my friends .Animals are my friends. And I don't eat my friends. Animals are my friends.*

And I don't eat my friends. Animals are my friends. And I don't eat my friends. Animals are my friends. And I don't eat my friends. Animals are my friends. And I don't eat my friends .Animals are my friends. And I don't eat my friends. Animals are my friends. And I don't eat my friends. Animals are my friends. And I don't eat my friends. Animals are my friends. And I don't eat my friends. Animals are my friends. And I don't eat my friends. Animals are my friends. And I don't eat my friends .Animals are my friends. And I don't eat my friends. Animals are my friends. And I don't eat my friends. Animals are my friends. And I don't eat my friends.

Animals are my friends. And I don't eat my friends. Animals are my friends. And I don't eat my friends .Animals are my friends. And I don't eat my friends. Animals are my friends. And I don't eat my friends. Animals are my friends. And I don't eat my friends. Animals are my friends. And I don't eat my friends. Animals are my friends. And I don't eat my friends .Animals are my friends. And I don't eat my friends. Animals are my friends. And I don't eat my friends. Animals are my friends. And I don't eat my friends. Animals are my friends. And I don't eat my friends. Animals are my friends. And I don't eat my friends. Animals are my friends. And I don't eat my friends .Animals are my friends. And I don't eat my friends. Animals are my friends. And I don't eat my friends. Animals are my friends. And I don't eat my friends. Animals are my friends. And I don't eat my friends. Animals are my friends. And I don't eat my friends. Animals are my friends. And I don't eat my friends .Animals are my friends. And I don't eat my friends. Animals are my friends. And I don't eat my friends. Animals are my friends. And I don't eat my friends. Animals are my friends. And I don't eat my friends. Animals are my friends. And I don't eat my friends. Animals are my friends. And I don't eat my friends .Animals are my friends. And I don't eat my friends. Animals are my friends. And I don't eat my friends. Animals are my friends. And I don't eat my friends. Animals are my friends. And I don't eat my friends. Animals are my friends. And I don't eat my friends. Animals are my friends. And I don't eat my friends .Animals are my friends. And I don't eat my friends. Animals are my friends. And I don't eat my friends. Animals are my friends. And I don't eat my friends. Animals are my friends. And I don't eat my friends. Animals are my friends. And I don't eat my friends. Animals are my friends. And I don't eat my friends .Animals are my friends. And I don't eat my friends. Animals are my friends. And I don't eat my friends. Animals are my friends. And I don't eat my friends. Animals are my friends. And I don't eat my friends. Animals are my friends. And I don't eat my friends. Animals are my friends. And I don't eat my friends. Animals are my friends.

The number of letters in last few pages, that is, around 7000, are the number of land animals slaughtered and killed before you finish counting 1,2, and 3.

CHAPTER 26

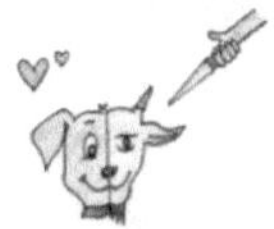

WHY PET SOME AND EAT OTHERS?

You have heard of racism, casteism, sexism, and other forms of discrimination. But have you heard about *Speciesism*?

Racism is to treat someone better or lower based on race. Casteism is to treat someone higher or lower based on caste. Sexism is discrimination with respect to gender. Speciesism, similarly, is a form of discrimination based on the species that the animal belongs to.

What is the difference between the love we have for our dog and any animal that is in a meat shop ready to be slaughtered?

Speciesism is treating members of one species as more important than members of other species even when their interests are equal.

Speciesism is a prejudice, bias, and partiality shown to animals in the same way bias shown to humans based on race, caste, or gender.

Speciesism is the first form of discrimination or bias that is taught at a young age. We were taught to love dogs and cats, but kill and eat chicken, goats, pigs, and were taught to steal from cows and hens.

All the animals, be it pets or ones that are killed for food, have hearts, brains, nervous systems, and the same capacity to suffer as we do. They may be different in certain ways like people who are different because of race, or caste, or gender.

If you claim that we pet dogs because they are intelligent, chickens, pigs, and cows are intelligent in their own way. It is just that we cannot see or understand their intelligence.

And, level of intelligence has nothing to do with the amount of love or compassion we should show to others. You do not discriminate because some one is less intelligent.

Loving animals and meat eating do not go together. "When we suffer, we suffer as equals and in their capacity to suffer, a dog is a pig is a bear is a boy" said Philip Wollen, an Australian philanthropist.

Speciesism, that is treating dogs and cats differently from chickens and goats, is no different from showing bias with respect to gender, nationality, religion, caste, or disability. And hence we should stop speciesism.

Recently an online poll asked us to choose the correct option:

(A) There is no difference between a DOG, CAT, CHICKEN, COW, or a PIG. Hence we should eat all of them.

(B) There is no difference between a DOG, CAT, CHICKEN, COW, or a PIG. Hence we should not eat any of them.

You can easily guess which one is correct. You cannot be an animal lover and meat eater at the same time. And that is final.

CHAPTER 27

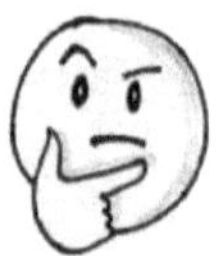

"FOOD IS MY PERSONAL CHOICE"

This is the last excuse most of us have – "food is my personal choice."

I have a personal choice to swing my arms and rotate as long as my arm does not hit the person standing next to me. If it hits, it is no more my personal choice.

Using polythene plastic bags is my personal choice. Why ban? I have a personal choice to smoke. Why ban in public? Driving petrol vehicles is my personal choice. Why plan to ban in future? Having babies is a personal choice. Why promote family planning?

We should respect the personal choice of everyone. We should respect the personal choice of 70 billion land animals and 3 trillion marine animals, who do not want to die but are killed every year against their will.

We are free to do what we want as long as it does not harm, exploit, or take away the rights and freedoms of others. Eating animals is not a personal choice since it is taking away the personal choice and freedom of animals to live. In addition, it is harming planet Earth and impacting everyone.

It is quite obvious that all animals or any living creature for that matter wants to live and sustain its species. Hence it is their personal choice to live.

Animals do have a personal choice. That is why animals run away when we try to harm or kill them. Ask your pet, dog or cat, if she or he wants to be sold and killed because your neighbor loves its meat?

Our freedom ends where others' freedom begins. We need to give animals a personal choice and a CHOICE to live. Hurting "others" is not a personal choice. And animals qualify as "others".

Caring about animals is not "optional". Making the issue *personal* is a nice way of saying "Don't hold me accountable for my actions that are harming animals."

Nature has designed non-human animals to have free will and freedom to choose like human animals.

Artificial breeding, exploitation, enslavement, killing, and profiteering from murder and selling corpses of 70 billion land animals and 3 trillion marine animals every year globally, devastating lives of animals, and impacting environment and lives of human beings is not a personal matter. If we do, it means we have institutionalized violence and legalized exploitation and murder.

"The ongoing atrocity against animals dwarfs all human atrocities combined," says Robert Grillo, an activist, author, and speaker for all species.

If you think eating meat just is a personal choice, you are forgetting someone who is an important co-traveler on earth.

"If you think that being vegan is difficult, imagine being a factory farmed animal" asks Davegan Raza.

CHAPTER 28

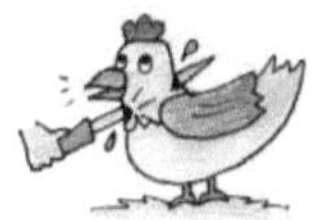

FREE RANGE, CAGE-FREE AND "HUMANE"!

There is no such thing as healthy cigarettes, healthy tobacco, or healthy alcohol. Similarly there is no cruelty-free meat, milk, dairy, or eggs.

You might have come cross these terms: free-range, freedom, organic, cage-free, antibiotic-free, hormone-free, grass-fed, buying-local, locally grown, "naatu" kozhi, and so on.

These are pure marketing terms, used to manipulate people to believe meat, dairy, or eggs can be produced in a humane or happy way. There is no such thing as humane murder and humane killing. There is no such thing as humane slavery, or humane harassment, or humane torture.

The public is becoming more aware of the daily horror that hens endure on factory egg farms. In response, the egg industry has created labels that sound appealing, such as "cage-free," "free-range," "free-roaming," "organic," and "natural" in order to attract more customers. But these labels are misleading. Here is something that the egg industry does not want you to know: "Cage-free" does not mean "cruelty-free."

Animals are living beings. From animals' point of view any one who commodifies and makes a business out of their body is brutal, cruel, and unforgivable.

Even if animals live extremely happy lives in free-range farms (which they do not), at the end of the day, they are going to be exploited or slaughtered for human use. This is where it is clear that free-range makes no sense at all. It is disguised cruelty. Say, you have a dog and you give him the best and comfiest life he could get, but you decide to send him to the slaughterhouse finally. Still cruel right? It is never humane to kill someone who does not want to die.

The health risk of getting diabetes, heart disease, osteoporosis, kidney problems, cancer, and other illnesses remain the same whether the meat, milk, and eggs are free-range, cage-free, grass-fed, organic, antibiotic-free, or hormone-free.

The USDA makes no claim that organically produced food is safer or more nutritious than conventionally produced food. "Organic, "natural," "humane," and "free-range" eggs, milk, and meat are filled with artery-clogging saturated fat and cholesterol, just like conventional meat, milk, and eggs.

Animal farming industry, namely, meat, dairy, and egg industries, thrive on your and my addiction to these products. All marketing strategies and communication strategies are used to keep this addiction intact and growing. Slaughter can never be humane when you are killing someone who does not want to die.

"Humane slaughter" does not cancel out the slaughter. It only cancels out your guilt. There is no humane way to kill someone who does not want to die.

The only truly humane foods are those that do not come from animals.

CHAPTER 29

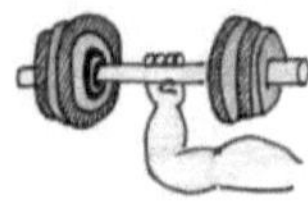

CAN VEGANS BE GAME CHANGERS?

You will be surprised to know that many athletes and sports persons who are well known today are vegans or vegetarians.

There is a huge list of vegans and vegetarian champions in sports. It proves that a plant-based diet avoiding meat and dairy can help you achieve in sports.

When going vegan, one thing that many people worry is about getting enough protein. Surprisingly, many great athletes and sports champions who eat plant-based food do not seem to be worried about getting enough protein. This is because they get plenty of healthy protein from plants.

Here is sample list of vegan sports people:

- Patrik Baboumian – body builder
- Venus Williams – tennis player
- David Haye – boxer
- Martina Navratilova – tennis player
- David Meyer – Brazillian jiu jitsu
- Scott Jurek – ultramarathon runner
- Sunil Chetri – Indian footballer
- Carl Lewis – Olympic Gold winner in athlete
- Novak Djokovic – tennis player

- Mac Danzig – mixed martial arts cage fighting
- Austin Aries – professional wrestling
- Lionel Messi – footballer
- Virat Kohli – Indian cricketer
- Chris Smalling – footballer
- Serena Williams – tennis player

American ultramarathon runner Scott Jurek who became vegan in 2000, set a record by running 266 kms in 24 hours in 2010.

Meet Kuntal Joisher, a mountaineer who accomplished the impossible – a 100-percent vegan ascent of the Mount Everest. "In 2018, he summited Mt. Lhotse, the fourth-highest mountain in the world at 8,516 m, and became the first person to ascend an 8,000 m mountain on a 100 percent vegan lifestyle. A year later, in 2019, he repeated the feat on Everest, another first for the vegan community," said a YourStory article.

Google "sports and vegan diet" and check out the facts yourself and your will be surprised.

"The Game Changers (2018)" is an eye-opening documentary film about the benefits of plant-based diet for athletes. It covers multiple success stories of plant-based athletes, references scientific studies, and touches on other arguments for plant-based diets.

This film was produced by Arnold Schwarzenegger (body builder, actor, and politician), Jackie Chan (martial artist and actor), James Cameron (Canadian filmmaker and director of Terminator), Lewis Hamilton (six-time Formula One world champion), Novak Djokovic (Ranked world No. 1 in men's singles tennis) , and Chris Paul (American professional basketball player).

'Game Changers' is available on Netflix or Prime Video. This is a must-watch documentary if you love sports.

CHAPTER 30

DOES FOOD IMPACT MIND AND THOUGHTS?

Every food item that we eat impacts both the body and the mind.

A very basic tenet of Ayurveda, a traditional Indian health system, is that food has a very strong impact on our mind and thoughts.

Sometimes it is evident (e.g, when one consumes alcohol) and its effects are visible. But, a lot of times it is subtle and requires keener observation. For example, if you eat food with a lot of spice, it makes you excited.

"What you eat directly affects the structure and function of your brain and, ultimately, your mood," says Eva Selhub, MD, in an article published by in Harvard Medical School. She continues, "Like an expensive car, your brain functions best when it gets only premium fuel. Unfortunately, just like an expensive car, your brain can be damaged if you ingest anything other than premium fuel."

According to Ayurveda, eating meat makes you more violent.

Based on the impact food has on one's mind, Ayurveda has divided food into three categories – sattvic, rajasic, and tamasic. Sattvic food brings peace of mind whereas rajasic food makes the mind excited and tamasic food makes one dull and angry.

Sattvic food is light and easy to digest, brings clarity in thinking, helps to unfold love and compassion, promotes the quality of forgiveness, and gives a feeling of contentment. Fresh vegetables, fruits, nuts, grains, legumes are examples of sattvic food.

Rajasic food is hot, spicy, and salty. All tempting foods come under rajasic category. Rajasic food makes mind more agitated and susceptible to temptations. A rajasic mind resorts to anger, hate, and manipulation. Chicken, fish, some vegetables like tamarind and broccoli, old sour milk, sour cream, hot pickles, and spicy chutneys that stimulate your mind are examples of rajasic foods.

Tamasic food is heavy, dull, and depressing. It induces dullness, lethargy, and sleep. Beef, lamb, pork, cheese, garlic, onion, and some grains like brown rice fall under tamasic food category.

Most of the food we eat should be plant-based and sattvic.

"Serotonin is a neurotransmitter that helps regulate sleep and appetite, mediate moods, and inhibit pain and about 95% of your serotonin is produced in your gastrointestinal tract," says Eva Selhub, MD. This proves what you are or what you think depends on what you eat.

Research has shown repeatedly that there is a strong correlation between mood and food. Nutritional psychiatry, a rapidly developing field, is finding there are many connections between what we eat, how we feel, and how we behave.

If you want your mind to be calm, composed, peaceful, and stress-free, then you should choose vegan diet.

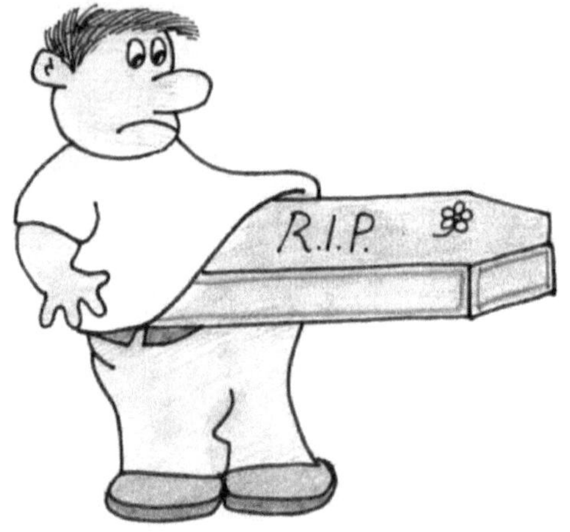

"Do not eat corpses and make your stomach their cemeteries."

CHAPTER 31

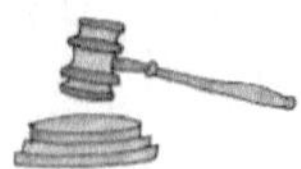

KICKING IS ILLEGAL. KILLING IS OK.

If you kill an animal, it is absolutely OK. But if you kick an animal you may be jailed and imprisoned for 3 months. Sounds wired? Yes. Welcome to Indian Act that deals with animals – The Prevention of Cruelty to Animals Act 1960 – and the connected ironies.

It is obvious that killing is cruel. Since this act permits and promotes the murder of animals, it should be ideally renamed as "The Killing and Murder of Animals Act." It is painful to see a law that permits killing of animals and on top of this, is named as "Prevention of Cruelty to Animals."

The Prevention of Cruelty to Animals Act 1960 does not make sense at all. As per The Prevention of Cruelty to Animals Act 1960, "if any person beats, kicks, overrides, overdrives, overloads, tortures or otherwise treats any animal so as to subject it to unnecessary pain or suffering...is punishable under the law."

But as you guessed it right, the mother of all torture – killing, slaughtering, slitting the throat, and so on – in the name of food – are permitted and you are well within the ambit of the law.

An Act that is so concerned about kicking and beating, happily permits killing of animals in slaughterhouses. The Act may say that animals are killed in such a way that there is no or minimum pain.

Will you accept if such law exists for human beings? The Act permits killing or destruction of animals if it does not inflict unnecessary pain or suffering.

Whether the animal so destructed did suffer unnecessary pain or not, only the animal can say. Only a victim can feel or vouch for the pain. How can others take a call that the victim did not suffer any pain?

Also, given the fact that, in India around 40 crores (400 million) of people are living on a vegetarian diet indicates that killing of animals for food, and hence inflicting pain and suffering, is unnecessary. Many medical experts have said repeatedly that animal products actually do more harm than good for human health. Hence killing animals is unnecessary.

Given the fact that the animal agriculture and slaughtering animals for food is causing enormous environmental destruction, killing animal is unnecessary.

We are not living in the Stone Age. We do not need to kill and eat animals to survive or to be healthy.

The whole purpose of this Act is defeated as it allows the extreme cruelty of killing the animals for food while there are plenty of plant-based food available for mankind. The Act has failed to see the fact that animals we slaughter for food are extremely intelligent and sensitive creatures. Killing of any animal is unnecessary and should be strictly banned by our legal system.

We are sure we all will evolve and will change our own shortsighted and "illegal" legal systems. As Peter Singer said, "Our future selves will consider slaughtering animals and meat eating to be barbaric."

CHAPTER 32

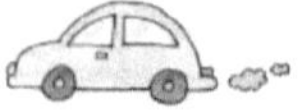

CARS ARE LESS DAMAGING FOR THE ENVIRONMENT!

Before cars... again few lines about food.

I thought food was always personal – that is, I do not have anything to say about what you eat OR you do not have anything to say about what I eat – until I read few insightful articles that surprised me on how what we eat impacts everybody else in the world, today, tomorrow, and for thousands of years to come.

"Meet the world's top destroyer of the environment. It is not the car, or the plane: it is the cattle. A United Nations report has identified the world's rapidly growing herds of cattle as the greatest threat to the climate, forests and wildlife," wrote *Independent UK* in December 2006.

An article by Care2, a social networking website, described "Cars are often used as the golden standard of environmental destruction. We know that our driving is hurtful to the environment."

But, what about a burger or biriyani containing meat? We don't normally associate meat consumption with climate change. But the dark side of the meat industry is worse and more damaging than cars when it comes to environment.

"University of Oxford found that, if everyone stopped eating meat and dairy products, global farmland use could be reduced by 75 per cent, an area equivalent to the size of the United States, China, Australia, and Europe combined. Not only would this result in a significant drop in greenhouse gas emissions, it would also free up wild land lost to animal agriculture, one of the primary causes for mass wildlife extinction," described another story in *Independent UK* in June 2018.

"Livestock emissions make up around 16 percent of total global greenhouse gas emissions. Comparably, the transportation sector is responsible for around 14 percent of emissions. By those numbers alone, our current system of meat production is extremely damaging. Perhaps more looming, however, is that while transportation creates CO2, livestock farming is hugely responsible for producing methane. As you may know, methane is 23 times more dangerous when it comes to warming the planet," elaborated Care2 .

"Giving up beef will reduce carbon footprint more than cars," described Guardian in a 2004 story.

Like you, I was shocked to learn that saving the earth starts from our plate, rather than cars.

* * *

If you are interested in learning more, my sincere suggestion is to watch *Cowspiracy*. *Cowspiracy* is a 2014 documentary film that explores the impact of animal agriculture on the environment. The film looks at various environmental concerns, including global warming, water use, deforestation, and ocean dead zones, and suggests that animal agriculture is the primary source of environmental destruction. Look for *Cowspiracy-Planet Climate Change* – full documentary on YouTube, which runs to about one and one half hour.

CHAPTER 33

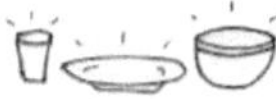

HALTING WORLD HUNGER

A total of 842 million are estimated to be suffering from chronic hunger, not getting enough food to conduct an active life regularly. Between now and 2050, the global population is projected to rise from about 7 billion to 9.2 billion, demanding a 60-percent increase in global food production according to a report from Food and Agriculture Organization (FAO), an arm of the United Nations.

You may be surprised to learn that halting the world hunger is driven by what we eat.

"Creating a hunger-free world is a major challenge for the world. But there is a solution: Cutting back on meat consumption could help end hunger by 2030. Today half the world's agricultural land is used for livestock farming, which is far less efficient for feeding people – and worse for the environment – than producing grains, fruits, and vegetables for direct human consumption," as per Huffington post.

World leaders are set to endorse a UN goal to eliminate hunger by 2030, but they will have to convince their citizens to adopt new eating habits first, experts say.

While being able to feed 70 billion land animals every year in the animal agriculture industry for meat and dairy, we are not able to feed 1 billion (800 million) people who are suffering from hunger. Ending hunger will require tough choices in the field and on the dinner table.

Let us move on to water. They have been saying the third world war will be about water. Water is becoming more and more scarce. Water scarcity is visible from California in the United States to Chennai in India.

It takes more than 20,000 liters of water to produce 1 kg of meat, while growing 1 kg of wheat requires just 200 liters of water.

Another statistics said, it takes 15,500 liters of water to produce 1 kg of beef, contrasted with 180 liters for 1 kg of tomatoes and 250 liters for 1 kg of potatoes.

An estimated 55% of the United States' freshwater supply goes to raising animals for food. Same will be true for other countries including India. It can take more than 600 liters of water to produce a single liter of cow's milk.

Consuming animal products is incredibly resource intensive, land intensive and water intensive.

Each day, humans worldwide drink an estimated 20 billion liters of water. Cows drink roughly eight and a half times that amount in a day – 170 billion litters.

A plant-based diet can save 4000 liters of water every day for each person, compared to a meat-based diet.

Check out here to know what water-friendly foods are: http://graphics.latimes.com/food-water-footprint/

CHAPTER 34

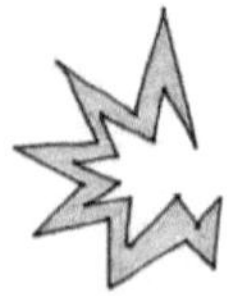

CAR CRASH IN SLOW MOTION?

What is the name for car crashing in slow motion? It is called "extinction." We need to be worried about this "slow-motion" car crash because you and I are the passengers inside the car!

There is a story in India about a frog accidently falling into a water bowl that is about to be kept on a stove for boiling. As the water gets warm, the frog enjoys the warmth without knowing what will happen in the next ten minutes. Similar is the state of us humans, who are overconsuming meat, dairy, and other resources without understanding what is in store for us in the next 20 to 200 years of time frame.

Our planet now faces a global extinction crisis never witnessed by humankind before. Scientists predict that more than 1 million species are on track for extinction in the coming decades.

According to research, at the current rate by 2050 (thirty years from now), 30 percent of all animal species will have disappeared from our planet. Another study says we will lose half of the existing land and marine species by 2100, that is, eighty years from now.

There have been five major extinctions in Earth's history one in 100 million years, on an average. The last mass extinction was 68 million years ago when a space rock fell on earth near Mexico, triggering a possible volcanic eruptions in India, wiping out dinosaurs and most of the land animals. But, don't worry, we humans were not there at that time! Humans came into existence just 2.5 million years ago and this extinction event was 60 million years ago!.

Scientist are predicting the sixth mass extinction is already in progress, though in slow motion and this time there is no space rock to blame! It is "we, humans!"

It is natural that many species go extinct and new species come into existence. But, what is worrying is the rate at which extinction is taking place and it is 1,000 to 3,000 times faster due to human activities.

Rapid growth of the human population is one of the key reasons for this ongoing mass extinction. Humans cause other species to become extinct by overharvesting, land clearing, overeating (of meat and dairy), hunting, overfishing, polluting, and changing forests into villages and later into towns and cities.

"We can put a person on the moon, we can come up with all these amazing technologies. We can reverse this in due time if we have the motivation. But what the data is showing is that we're not doing that. We're putting our foot further on the pedal," said marine biologist David Gruber.

It would likely take several millions of years of normal evolutionary diversification to restore the Earth's species to what they were prior to humans.

Time to go vegan yet?

CHAPTER 35

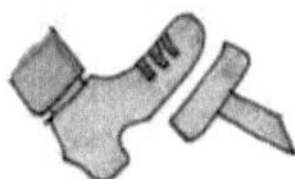

STOPPING THE CAR CRASH

If we continue to exploit the resources of the planet, like the way we do now, one day even our human race might become extinct sooner than we think. The Earth is already becoming less conducive to all living beings including humans, due to harmful and excessive human activities as evidenced by global warming, climate change, and pandemics.

One third of all animal and plant species on the planet could face extinction by 2070 due to climate change, a new study warns.

Animals, wildlife, and plants are the foundation on which our human lives are built and revolve around.

Jonas Salk, an American physician, medical researcher, and virologist, famously said, "If all insects on Earth disappeared, within 50 years life on earth would end. If all human beings disappeared from earth, within 50 years all forms of life would flourish."

Though we are all busy and obsessed with noise and speed of modern urban life, we still have deep connection, both physically and emotionally to animals, wildlife, and plants.

"Across cultures, humans inherently value nature. The magic of seeing fireflies flickering long into the night is immense. We draw energy from nature. We find sources of food, medicine, livelihoods, and innovation in nature. Our well-being fundamentally depends on nature," says Achim Steiner, an environmentalist and an administrator at UNDP.

In addition, the presence of wildlife, animals, and trees bring joy to us. That is why we take a break and go for vacation or go for a trek in the forest.

However, the current extinction of animals, plants, and insects will make our home (earth) a very lonely place for us and our future generations.

Scientists find billions of populations of mammals, birds, reptiles, and amphibians have already been lost, all over the planet, in the last 200 years.

Going vegan, avoiding animal products for food such as meat and dairy, stopping animal breeding and agriculture, ending fishing, using fewer fossil fuels, driving less frequently, not disturbing wildlife, reducing overall consumption and recycling are some of means to slow the rate of extinctions.

Reducing water usage and refraining from using herbicides and pesticides can also protect local wildlife.

Unlike the mass extinction events of geological history, the current extinction challenge is one for which a single species, ours, appears to be almost wholly responsible.

"When we lose an animal species to extinction, we lose part of our family," says Anthony Douglas.

Hence we should get our act together and stop the car crash.

CHAPTER 36

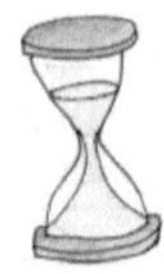

FOR A MOMENT OF TASTE

As they sit around the table,
Happy as they could be
Dinner was served as tasty as it could be.

Just that morning the sheep was stabbed to death
And the hen's throat was sliced up within a single breath

Just that morning the calf was dragged from his mother.
The cows saw helplessly as he died. They had lost their brother.

The family smile to one another as joyous as ever
And start eating the meal that was as sumptuous as ever

Just that noon the chicken helplessly moaned as her throat was severed.
Just that noon the humans sneered as the goat's life was severed.

Not one knew that for a moment of taste
They had laid complete waste
To innocent beings that just wanted to live,
Though in vain
They had all died in pain.

Peace is what we cry for

Helheim on earth is what we've brought.
Murder and bloodshed is what we've got.
Understand we must, that Thanatos we're not.

Humane we justify
Yet animals we crucify.

Peace is what we cry for
But animals we've murdered so far.
Is this the world we aspire to live on?

Joyful Hell

As I step into his deadly realm
I scream and cry as the pains overwhelm
In the blood stained lands overrun by elms
I lay in the treachery of woeful elves.

Caged lay I, never to see but plight
For crumbled lay my hope and light.

He claims he's humane
Yet by murder and pain, is the bane
Of earth as he wanes all of life

Then I step into the gruesome hell
And see boundless joy as far as I could tell.

(The life of animals at slaughter house is worse than hell.
Hell is joyful compared to a slaughter house).

Poems by Manish, a student and an animal lover.

CHAPTER 37

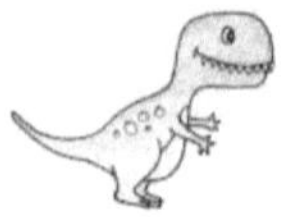

NATURE'S EXPERIMENT?

"Nature is a great experimenter," says Preetha Ji of PK Consciousness. She continues:

"Nature is constantly experimenting over millions of years. It evaluates and discards the species that is not supporting the whole.

It has discarded dinosaurs, Saber tooth tigers, Ramapithecus, and Neanderthals. A few of these species have survived for 200,000 years. A few of them have also survived for 10 to 20 million years. (Humans have been around for 2.5 million years.)

But the question is, how sure are we about the success of our species, the humans? Are you sure we are going to survive forever? If we have to survive forever, we need to be beneficial for the whole. If we are not going to be beneficial for the whole, what would nature do? It would discard us.

Are we being beneficial to the whole? If you have a conversation with planet Earth, what do you think planet Earth will tell us? It would say I am very unhappy with humans.

We are probably more damaging than the smallpox virus, which does not exist now. We are very damaging, causing greater calamity and being cruel to this planet of ours and its inhabitants. If you look at other species, every other species kills somebody else or kills another species only for its own survival, only when it is threatened, or when it is very hungry.

But, as a human species, we have not evolved. We as a species, kill another species, not for our own survival, but to prove our superiority over the others, to prove our dominance over this entire planet Earth, and many times even for pleasure.

There is a huge noise in the world about the coronavirus. What if the coronavirus is nature's way of eliminating 'the human virus', which is causing endless harm to planet Earth?

There is a huge possibility, right? If we are not being beneficial to the whole, we have seen, that nature will eliminate us soon.

China is not the problem. Chinese people are not the problem. What is the problem? The problem is our own mindset. We are living life in separation and experiencing life as though we are separate from every living thing around us and as though we are superior.

This mindset has its own repercussions and we see it in the world. We see it in the world as cancer, as disaster, as natural calamity or as the coronavirus now. It is time to wake up. If you are truly looking for a more peaceful and a more joyful world, if we intend to create a beautiful world for our children and grandchildren, then the transformation has to happen now and here. It is already too late."

CHAPTER 38

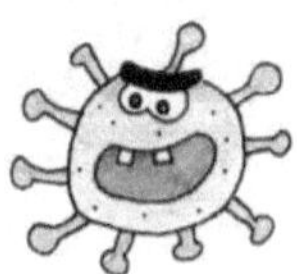

CARNIVOROUS AND CORONAVIRUS

"Dear God, could you please uninstall 2020 and re-install it? It has a virus!" said a social media post.

Millions of people got infected, thousands died, many became critically ill across countries due to coronavirus.

Coronavirus or COVID-19 comes after SARS (severe acute respiratory syndrome in 2003) and MERS (Middle East respiratory syndrome in 2012).

While MERS came from camels and SARS from civet cats, coronavirus has come from pangolins. It is not of significance if these animals have infected the virus from bats or rats or cats.

Many coronaviruses are zoonotic diseases, and they spread from animals to people.

The COVID-19 outbreak has originated at a live-animal market in Wuhan in China, and illegal pangolin trade is the key cause for coronavirus outbreak.

* * *

Pangolins are shy nocturnal animals usually found in Asia and Africa and they are ant eaters. They are mammals and are the most trafficked mammals in the world.

There is global ban on trading Pangolins, but, China remains a major trading spot for pangolins. Pangolins , are killed for their meat and scales for Chinese medicine.

From 2000 until 2013, it is estimated that more than a million pangolins are killed and sold in the illegal markets.

Despite the ban, between 2016 and 2019, about 200+ tons of pangolin scales were seized in China. And this number is official and you can guess the actual numbers.

On top of all of these, it is sad to learn that all existing pangolin species are nearing extinction; many of the Asian species of pangolins are listed as critically endangered. But still we humans kill them in thousands (250 thousands) every year.

Rare and endangered animals are sold openly in wildlife markets in China, such as Wuhan wildlife markets. The price list in one of the shops read – body parts of camels, koalas and birds, live wolf pups, golden cicadas, scorpions, bamboo rats, squirrels, foxes, civets, porcupines, salamanders, turtles, and crocodiles.

Death of thousands of people was required to permanently ban wildlife trade in China. How many more deaths will be required to ban trading of animals in general? Lives of animals and people are equally precious and we should find ways to avoid pandemics such as this one. One way is to stop eating animals and opting for plant-based food.

Carnivorous and Coronavirus are incidentally anagrams, that is, a word formed by rearranging the letters of another word. On the other hand, "veganism" and "saving me" are anagrams as well.

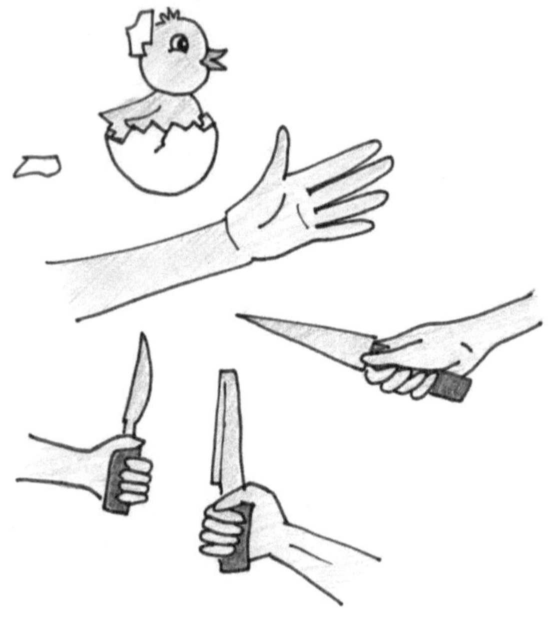

What a crazy society we
live in, where we have to
explain why killing
animals is wrong.

CHAPTER 39

STOPPING THE NEXT PANDEMIC

Covid-19 pandemic made us locked up in our own homes, like animals in the zoo.

In keeping ourselves busy and with the overwhelming news and videos, during lockdown, we have forgotten one important thing – the root cause of COVID-19 or the current coronavirus.

The coronavirus did not come from the moon, neither did it travel from Mars. Coronavirus is an earthly creation.

How did we humans get infected with coronavirus? Did we get infected with coronavirus by eating potato or tomato, banana or mango, greens or grains?

With the outbreak of the coronavirus, which has originated from a wet meat market, isn't it time to think about ways to prevent future pandemics?

The next virus can come from a wet market in our own city or an Indian poultry farm or an American slaughterhouse? It can come from anywhere. The problem came because of our interference with the lives of animals for our food and selfish needs.

India's poultry industry currently sells 95% of its product through wet markets, fresh food markets where animals are sold live and then processed either onsite or in the consumer's home. These wet markets pose numerous sanitary risks as well.

The New York Times reported in May 2020, "An astonishing six out of 10 counties that the White House itself identified as coronavirus hot spots are home to the very slaughterhouses the US government ordered to open. The Smithfield pork plant, which produces some 5 percent of the country's pork, is one of the largest hot spots in the nation. A Tyson plant in Perry, Iowa, had 730 cases of the coronavirus – nearly 60 percent of its employees. At another Tyson plant, in Waterloo, Iowa, there were 1,031 reported cases among about 2,800 workers."

People feel it's okay to eat the animals they eat, but they are not okay with other humans eating the animals they don't eat, in this case Chinese eating pangolins or bats.

"Honestly, there is no difference between eating a chicken, cow, goat, pigs, or camels and eating dogs, bats, civets, snakes, raccoon dogs, or porcupines. They are all animals slaughtered for food in different cultures," says vegan activist Sharmila Shanmugasundaram.

If you want to stop the next pandemic, we should stop eating animals and meat – be it cows, goats, chickens, pigs, dogs, cats, frogs, pangolins, or bats. All governments in all countries should ban slaughterhouses and sale of meat.

By eating meat, we are creating stress to the earth. We are putting millions or billions of animals – who have similar feelings, emotions, and ability to feel pain – into murder and endless torture.

Humans can very well survive, thrive, and be healthy and happy on a plant-based lifestyle.

CHAPTER 40

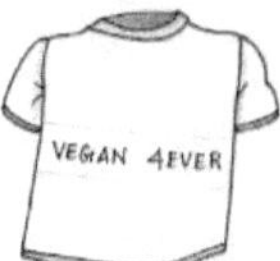

COMPASSIONATE CLOTHING

You would be surprised to learn that the clothes we wear and the washing machines we use - are harming animals and marine animals to be specific. If meat is killing land animals and causing annihilation, the materials we use for clothing and the way we wash our clothes are killing marine animals slowly.

One primary source of ocean pollution impacting large number of marine animals has mainly remained unnoticed so far – and that's microfiber. Microfiber consists of microscopic bits of polyester, acrylic, and nylon from our clothes that come out during washing cycles.

Every time we run our washing machine, hundreds of thousands of microfibers are flushed down the drain. Much of these microfibers reach oceans where they remain for hundreds of years, being swallowed by fish and other sea animals, impacting their health and life. One piece of clothing can release 700,000 microfibers in a single wash.

Microfibers, most commonly made from polyesters, that is, essentially made of plastic, are now used in about 60% of our clothes.

"Your car has filters, your washing machine should have them too. Every washing machine should be neutral to the environment," says Mojca Zupan, founder of PlanetCare.

If we take into account the fossil fuels used in the production of polyester clothing, CO_2 emissions of polyester clothing are nearly three times higher than that of cotton.

Our dependence on polyester is one of the reasons for pollution. Polyester making is emissions-heavy and non-biodegradable waste-heavy.

It is not just the marine animals. Micro plastic travels through the food chain and ends up on our plates as well. A research says we are eating one credit card size of plastic every year and this is growing each year.

Clothes should be produced and used without polluting the environment. It may not be easy to get rid of synthetic fibers altogether, but we should start with buying less. We shop and stack too much of clothes. As per a survey, about 50% of our clothes are rarely or never worn. Why over-buy?

Clothing made from plant-based materials is environmentally superior to polyester or petroleum-based clothing. Cotton and plant-based clothing prevents microfibers and plastic pollution.

In addition to microfibers from clothing, oceans also have plastic pollution arising from discarded plastic bags, cups, and bottles, impacting sea life. Hence we should reduce use of plastics, especially single-use plastics such as water bottles, straws, foam plates, foam cups, plastic cups, and polythene bags.

In addition to food, it is time to understand how what we wear and what we use are impacting the environment. Use of plant-based clothing and plant-based materials is clearly good for long-term health of marine animals, the oceans, our earth, and our own health.

CHAPTER 41

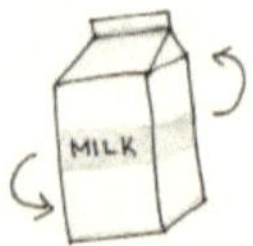

FREEDOM FROM MILK CYCLE

Kitchen work and chores are already tedious. Every person in the kitchen, would love to get rid of the "milk cycle" that is integral part of kitchen, if given a chance.

Here is a story from an Indian woman who liberated herself from complex milk cycle, by turning vegan.

"We used to buy milk in packets, which comes in different colors with different jargons printed on it such as homogenized, standardized, and pasteurized, which I had never really understood.

We used to pay the milk vendor a month in advance and adjust the amounts for the days when we either don't buy milk or get lesser than usual quota or get extra milk packets, in the next month's payment.

A basket was fixed outside our home almost permanently to enable the milk vendor, who comes as early as 4:30 am, to deliver milk. When we travel outstation and do not need milk or when we need lesser quantity, I had to set up a process of keeping a placard in the basket, the day before, saying "No milk," "1 Packet only" or "Extra 2 Packets" and so on, which I later upgraded into a WhatsApp communication.

Planning all this along with other chores is not easy, especially, if you are a working woman.

In the morning, even before you open your eyes, you need to open the door, take the milk packets and keep them inside the refrigerator; otherwise the milk will soon turn bad, especially in a tropical climate such as ours in India.

Even inside the fridge, you need to have a separate process for the milk because there will be previous day's leftover milk, which should not get mixed with that day's new milk.

Boiling milk without getting it spilt is both science as well as art! It will not even give a sign of boiling as long as you are close to it! But when you step out for few seconds, it will promptly boil and spill all over the gas stove, giving you heart burns. Also half of the milk would have gone down the drain!

You also need to make curd or yogurt. Boiled milk needs to be brought to room temperature and then we have to ferment it with a spoonful of yogurt. South Indian meals always end with "thayir sadam," that is, rice with yogurt. You need to keep the yogurt inside the fridge next day morning without forgetting; otherwise, you are in for a "sour" surprise.

Then, you also separate the yellowish layer or cream from the yogurt and collect it. Once a week, as a modern day Yashodha, you churn this to get butter and butter milk. Part of butter, we usually melt it and make ghee, which is used with rice, roti, or bread.

I was stuck in the cycle of milk-yogurt-butter-butter milk-ghee for many years, until one day, for reasons of compassion toward animals, I went vegan. I liberated the cows from artificial insemination, hormone injections, milking machines, and cruel treatment and liberated myself from the milk cycle as well. How free and great it feels!"

CHAPTER 42

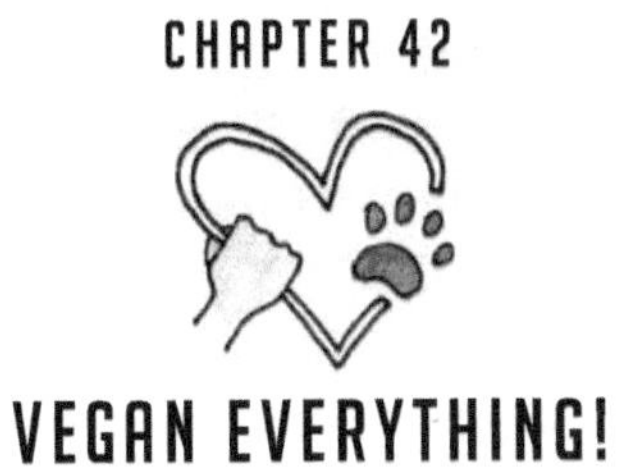

VEGAN EVERYTHING!

Though on one hand we are chained by a habit of being cruel to animals and consuming animal products, there is a silver lining in the sky.

The world is rapidly adopting veganism. As much as 25% of people in the age group of less than 30 years in the United States have declared themselves as vegans. In the same age group, 28% of people are vegans in the United Kingdom, as per the data shown in a vegan conference held in 2019.

Because of this new-found awareness, many things are going the vegan way.

<u>Vegan food</u>: Companies like Beyond Meat and Tofurkey in the United States are producing mass-market pea-based protein and tofu-based products designed to replace animal protein.

<u>Vegan beauty</u>: Beauty Without Cruelty is a British company that manufactures vegan cosmetics, which contain no animal products and are not tested on animals.

Body Shop, a UK-based company, manufactures vegan cosmetics, which contain no animal products, and are not tested on animals. Kinder Beauty Box by Evanna Lynch (Harry Potter actress) and Florance By Mills by Millie Bobby Brown (Stranger Things actress) are vegan and cruelty free.

<u>Vegan cars</u>: CEO of Tesla, Elon Musk, told shareholders that the Model 3 and the Model Y would be fully vegan by 2020. Now, he has officially fulfilled his promise on the former.

<u>Vegan temple</u> : A Jain temple in California, United States, is the world's first vegan and ahimsa temple and it does not use or serve dairy and animal products.

<u>Vegan apps</u> : Happy Cow is an app (like Swiggy or Zomato) for discovering vegan restaurants and plant-based foods globally.

<u>Vegan city</u>: London (UK) is the vegan capital of the world where you find more vegan food and vegan products than any other city. Other vegan-friendly cities include New York (USA), Bristol (UK), Berlin (Germany), Tel Aviv (Israel), and Portland (USA).

<u>Vegan clothing</u>: Clothing made from plant-based materials are environmentally superior to polyester or petroleum-based clothing. Cotton and plant-based clothing prevents microfibers and plastic pollution.

<u>Vegan schools</u>: The German International School, Chennai is first 100% vegan school in India. The students learn about veganism and the school serves only plant-based foods. "When all the evidence is added up, it no

longer makes sense to serve meat for children. The only way to be a truly 'green and compassionate' community is to choose veganism," says the school. MUSE School in California in the United States is another vegan school.

There are also vegan families, vegan couples, vegan communities, who are recognizing the need for going vegan. What we need now is a vegan world.

CHAPTER 43

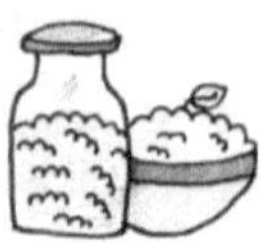

SAUERKRAUT AND VEGURT RICE

If you are a vegan and worried about probiotics, it is time to turn to sauerkraut!

Wondering what sauerkraut is?

When life gives you lemons make lemonade and when life gives you cabbages make sauerkraut or kraut. Sauerkraut, a German dish, is cabbage fermented in salt water, as simple as that.

All you need to do is to prepare shredded cabbage and some salt and pack it into a container. The cabbage releases a liquid and creates its own brine or salt solution. You need to leave this for a period of several days or weeks and the cabbage slowly ferments into the crunchy, sour condiment, which goes by the name sauerkraut.

Sauerkraut fermentation creates conditions that promote the growth of beneficial probiotics, similar to those that you find in yogurt.

Sauerkraut is rich in probiotics, vitamins, fiber, and minerals, which can contribute to better digestion and a stronger immune system.

Sauerkraut, like pickles, goes well with sandwiches, roti, or breads and can be used as a side dish for any food that we have.

If you are a vegan from the southern part of India, and used to eat curd rice every day, no worries! Vegurt or "vegan yogurt" rice is coming to your help. Here is a quick recipe.

Just cook fresh rice in the night. Then cool it down and add water to the cooked rice and soak it overnight. Instead of fresh rice, you may also use cooked rice that is left over from lunch.

Then on the next day morning, after 8 to 10 hours of soaking, remove the excess water. Now smash the rice a bit and add salt, a dash of lemon, seasoned mustard and garnish with green chilies, bit of ginger, and top it with coriander leaves. You have wonderful vegurt rice ready.

This slightly fermented humble breakfast is refreshing and cooling. It is rich in vitamins, vitamin B12 in specific, and iron. It cures stomach ulcers and prevents you from dehydration during summers.

Yogurt rice also can be made from peanut yogurt made from peanut milk.

* * *

The above are examples of few recipes out of millions out there with which you can happily and easily lead a life without torturing and killing animals and avoiding meat, milk, eggs, and dairy in your menu.

Surf the Internet to explore many interesting vegan recipes. Thousands of easy-to-make vegan recipes are just a click away.

CHAPTER 44

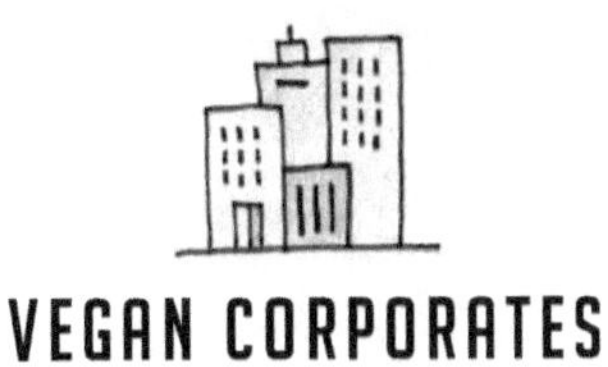

VEGAN CORPORATES

Many businesses including multinational organizations are increasingly adopting a vegan policy given the enhanced sensitivity to animals, environment, health, and climate change.

Forbes, in 2018, reported, "Vegan initiatives are taking off in the corporate workplace and it's good for business."

For example, New York-based WeWork, $20 billion startup, went vegetarian citing environmental concerns.

WeWork, which has built its business around shared workspaces, has done away with meat and poultry from corporate dining functions. The company of around 6,000 will no longer serve meat at events or reimburse employees for pork, red meat or poultry, as per EcoWatch.

Another London-based company Playtypus has adopted climate-friendly vegan food policy.

Vegan Leaders in Corporate Management – VLCM (http://veganleaders.com/), a global community for vegans working in corporate functions, continues to grow quickly and expansively. It has more than 4000 members, including those from Google, Boeing, Amazon, Intel, and Accenture.

As per Forbes, Facebook and Dropbox have seen successful employee-driven vegan initiatives. Dropbox has embraced a vegan employee program called "Vegbox," turning it into a vibrant vegan meal and sustainability platform for employees.

People working in large corporates like Microsoft, IBM, GE, and Tesla are increasingly embracing vegan policies at work.

At HelloLeads (www.HelloLeads.io), a CRM software product company, in which I have been part of, we have gone vegetarian, as a step toward vegan journey.

Organizations can follow below polices:

- Food sponsored by organizations to customers, government representatives or business guests, by the company shall be vegan.
- Food expenses of employees borne by the company while traveling or during outstation business trips will be for vegetarian or vegan food only.
- During team meetings or annual events, organizations can go with vegan food.
- Employees can be encouraged to bring vegan lunch.
- Organizations can show enhanced sensitivity to animals, environment, health, and climate change as part of their business culture.

Business leaders who are vegan include Twitter co-founder Biz Stone, MIT Media Lab Director Joi Ito, Ford

Executive Chairman Bill Ford Jr., Canadian media tycoon Mort Zuckerman, Binatone founder and chairman Gulu Lalvani, Wynn Resorts CEO Steve Wynn, and Eleveneleven's Ellen Degeneres. The list is endless and there are many more.

CHAPTER 45

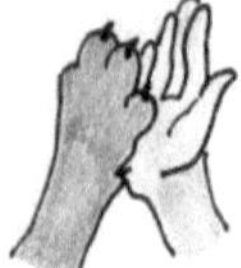

HUMAN AND NON-HUMAN ANIMALS

When I ask people what is the difference between humans and animals, they say animals have five senses and humans have six senses, indirectly meaning humans are superior to animals.

This is an incorrect way of representation "designed" to purely exploit animals for our selfish reasons.

Common sense and many scientific studies show that there are many things that animals can do which we cannot. We cannot fly like birds, let alone fly like a bat with eyes closed. We cannot find our way back in a new city, forget getting back home across continents like a migratory bird. Animals have their own sixth sense suiting their environment and needs.

Plants, animals, humans – we are all in one continuum and there is no real difference between any adjacent species in evolution. We need to remind ourselves that we are oxygen-breathing biped mammals and animals. If you recollect school-day biology lessons, humans are classified under "animal kingdom". Hence, it will be more precise to categorize the animal kingdom as human animals and non-human animals.

Human animals are not superior to non-human animals and we have no right to think that we are more evolved and thus have right to kill and exploit non-human animals.

If we, human animals, rule over other non- human animals, our days can be numbered. Studies show that dinosaurs struggled for millions of years before the asteroid impact. Fossils from around the world suggest the terrible lizards were in decline before the collision.

"We are not special, we were not placed here by a God to be the custodians of the Earth and if we were, we have let the Almighty down big time!" read an article.

It is a myth and "human-centric" assumption that we, human animals, are special and that we will continue to live forever as a dominant species.

If we continue to do what we do, we will be wiped out over a period of time and other, more adaptable, life forms will take our place. Poet John Donne wrote: "Do not ask for whom the bell tolls, it tolls for thee."

* * *

The earth is 4500 million years old. Life started 3500 million years ago on earth. Animals came into existence around 600 million years ago. Mammals came into existence some 160 million years ago. Great apes (chimpanzees, gorillas, and orangutans) came into existence 20 million years ago. Humans came into existence 2.5 million years ago. Anatomically modern humans or *Homo sapiens* came into existence 1 million years ago.

If you think the age of earth is a year or 365 days, then anatomically modern humans or *Homo sapiens*, we are here on earth for less than 2 hrs! We need to know how recent we are to this place and hence should stay humble and take care of our "pre-existing" co-travelers. Should not we?

CHAPTER 46

LEARNING COMPASSION

In June 2005, a twelve-year-old girl was kidnapped by four men in rural south-west Ethiopia when she was returning from school. She was terrified. A week after kidnapping, when the men were attempting to move her to a new place in the forest, three lions attacked the men and chased the men off and started protecting the girl.

The lions remained with the terrified girl, almost for six hours, till police officers located her and escorted her to safety.

Police say they found the girl "shocked and terrified" – and surrounded by lions. The massive animals quickly dispersed when officers arrived. She told them that although she had been beaten by her kidnappers – who it is believed had been attempting to sell her into a forced marriage – the lions had not touched her.

Sergeant Wondmu Wedaj of Ethiopia said, "They stood guard until we found her and then they just left her like a gift and went back into the forest."

* * *

Gorillas are extremely dangerous animals protecting their territory. They do not allow anyone to come near them either in the wild or in zoos (zoos are non-vegan, by the way, as they cage animals).

At Brookfield Zoo in Illinois, in 1996, when a 3-year-old boy accidentally fell into the gorilla enclosure, zoo employees anticipated the worst. Giant gorillas can disfigure and even kill full-grown men – so you can imagine the damage they are capable of inflicting on a small child.

After the little boy fell in, Binti, a 7-year-old female gorilla ran over to the boy and picked him up. Then, she carried him carefully to the door of the cage, so that rescue workers could retrieve him. Binti handed over the boy safely.

* * *

Snakes eat frogs for food. In Sringeri, a forest area in Karnataka (India), one thousand years ago, during a very hot summer, a pregnant frog was struggling in the hot sun and was about to give birth to babies. But the hot sun would have killed the frog and the eggs. A cobra who was passing by, seeing this, came near the frog, raised his hood and protected the frog from the hot sun. The snake gave shade to the frog as the frog was undergoing labour pains.

Adi Sankara, a saint, witnessed this with his own eyes and recoded the story and how animals are compassionate. As a piece of evidence to this, today, one can see a sculpture called Kappe Shankara on the footsteps to the river Tunga, in Sringeri.

Animals are capable of compassion, kindness, and altruism. They are known to step in and save those weaker than themselves at the most unexpected of times, and in ways that humans often fail to predict.

It is time we humans exhibit our compassion and kindness towards animals by refraining from killing and eating them or torturing them. It is time for humans to learn compassion from animals.

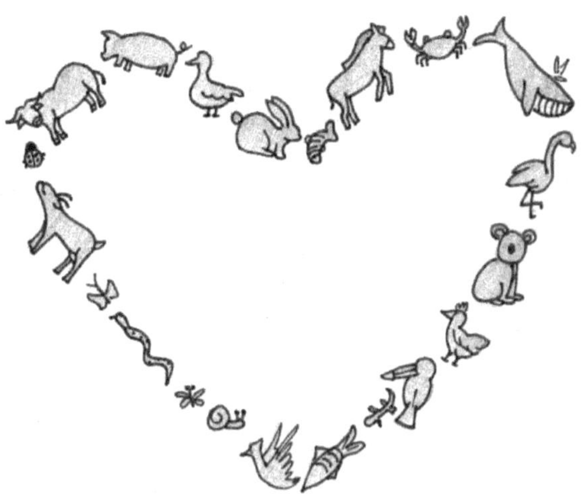

"A person doesn't
have two hearts,
One for animals and
another for humans.

One either has a heart
or one doesn't."

Alphone de Lamartine
French Poet

CHAPTER 47

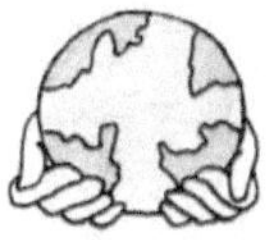

VEGAN OR WE'RE GONE...

We are running out of time, if you notice.

We have been killing, murdering, and massacring animals without thinking even a bit. It is having a huge impact on animals, environment, climate, and our earth.

Blame it on tradition, habit, taste, and addiction – 70 billion land animals and 3 trillion marine animals are killed and consumed every year by us.

If we make a line of 70 billion land animals, it will come around earth 532 times! "Where is the kind hearted part of us?" "Where has that animal lover in you gone?"

Around 30 percent of the earth's ice-free land is used for livestock production, as per UN, and livestock production generates nearly 20% of world's greenhouse gases – more than cars and transportation.

Cruelty and over consumption are killing animals and the planet. Food is the next nuclear bomb and it is already exploding, disguised in slow-motion.

We were all born vegan. We loved animals when we were children and would never let anyone kill an animal in front of our eyes. That is why there are no school trips to slaughterhouses. We were blindfolded and in the name of tradition, habit, and culture were made addicted to meat and dairy.

If we are able to feed 70,000 million land animals every year, why are not we able to feed 800 million people who suffer from hunger and malnutrition? The majority of grains grown in the world feeds cattle, cows, pigs, and chickens, which are artificially produced and bred to satisfy human palate and greed.

We are in the midst of the sixth mass extinction because of overuse of land, animal agriculture, overfishing, water shortage, and pollution arising from excessive animal farming.

It is time to move on to veganism. Stop eating meat, cheese, milk, and eggs. Move on to a fully plant-based diet and life.

As already proven, plant-based food is more than sufficient to live well. Plants are the only original source of protein on earth and has vitamins, minerals, and amino acids. Medical science has proven animal protein is a major cause for diabetes, heart diseases, cancer, osteoporosis, and many other health issues.

We hear many excuses starting from animals do not suffer, plants also feel pain, lions eat meat, it is the circle of life, meat has protein, and so on. They are meaningless and make no sense if we think with our heart and mind.

Food is no more a personal choice as what we eat impacts animals' right to live, impacts generations to come, and all people living on planet Earth. It is time we place the planet before our palate.

Vegan or we're gone!

CHAPTER 48

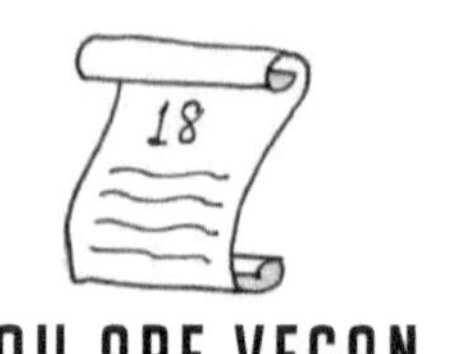

IF YOU ARE VEGAN ...

If you are vegan, you take care of 18 things listed below:

1) You respect the right of animals to live, just like how humans have the right to live.

2) You stop exploiting animals. You understand animals have emotions, have feelings, and can feel pain just like you and I do.

3) You follow a kind, compassionate, and ahimsa way of life and living.

4) You do not eat animals of any kind – be it chicken, fish, goats, pigs, or cows.

5) You do not eat eggs because hens are caged, crammed, and exploited.

6) You do not consume milk or dairy products since cow's milk is for baby cows and cows are exploited in the process of obtaining milk.

7) You do not consume products that contain dairy – chocolates, ice-creams, paneer, butter, ghee, or cheese.

8) You live happily and healthily by eating plant-based food.

9) You do not use leather or leather products because animals are murdered for obtaining leather. There has been so much scientific advancement in

material science and it is a shame to depend on animal skins, the way we did in stone ages.

10) You do not use silk. Approximately 3000 worms are killed (boiled alive at cocoon stage) to get one meter of silk thread.

11) You do not use honey as honeybees need honey for their survival. We steal honey from them and honey bees are exploited.

12) You use beauty products that are free from animal ingredients and those that are not tested on animals.

13) You do not use woolen or fur materials.

14) You do not encourage zoos or circuses since they use, captivate, cage, and harm animals. They interfere in the freedom of animals.

15) You discourage the use of animals for scientific experiments and medical testing.

16) You say no to hunting, fishing, bullfighting, cockfighting, and other entertainments that involve or use animals.

17) You do not visit temples or places of religious worship where animals are sacrificed.

18) You adopt and embrace a vegan way of living because it helps animals and also you to live peacefully.

CHAPTER 49

IDEAS THAT WE SHOULD LOOK AT

Ideas for saving the animals, earth, and ourselves:

<u>Education</u>: Introduce lessons on animal rights, veganism, and climate change for school children – say in grades or standards 3, 5 and 7. Projects and assignments should be given to students, which should focus on compassion and equal rights to animals.

Have a subject, like history and geography, veganism and animal rights in grade or standard 9. Have a subject on veganism, animal rights, and climate change for MBBS, nutritional science, and students of appropriate streams.

<u>Food</u>: Have vegan label for food products. Introduce a yellow dot in addition to red and green. Red for meat, yellow for vegetarian, and green for vegan.

Ask restaurants to have mandatory vegan menu. Food provided by government, be it noon meal scheme, corporation-run food outlets, or food in prisons need to be vegan—no meat, dairy, or eggs. Menu prescribed by hospitals and doctors need to be vegan.

<u>Tax and subsides:</u> Tax meat, fish, milk, and dairy more so that it compensates for the damage they are causing to earth and animals. Provide subsides for vegan and

organic products because it will help to improve the environment in the long run.

<u>Law:</u> Stop animal sacrifice in the name of religion, immediately. Celebrate religious holidays in nonviolent, compassionate ways. Say no to animal sacrifice.

Do away with zoos and circuses using animals. Increase forests, natural habitats over a period of time.

Stop chicken farms and animal farms and slaughter houses. Regulate and gradually decrease sale of meat and animal products.

Stop trading of animals (selling and buying, transporting) in the next 5 years. Ban slaughterhouses and wet markets and ban sale of meat and animal products fully within the next 10 years.

<u>Commerce and products:</u> Introduce a label for "Cruelty Free" similar to ISI, which indicates beauty products and medicines were not tested on animals. Also include labels on meat products, such as "This was made by killing an animal who didn't want to die."

Ban import and export of animal products including meat, dairy, leather, medicines, or cosmetics that involve animal-based ingredients.

<u>Materials</u>: Eliminate one-time-use plastics and microfiber-generating clothing to save marine animals.

<u>Communication:</u> Encourage movies and documentaries on veganism. Government and schools should screen

Saivam a Tamil movie, *Game Changers, Cowspiracy,* and other similar movies in public places.

<u>Society:</u> Create skills and alternate employment opportunities for people in meat and dairy industry.

CHAPTER 50

MUST-READ BOOKS

Below are few books that you may want to read to learn more about compassion for animals and how palate, plates, and planet are interconnected.

A Plea for the Animals
The Moral, Philosophical, and Evolutionary Imperative to Treat All Beings with Compassion
Matthieu Ricard

The China Study
The Most Comprehensive Study of Nutrition Ever Conducted
T. Colin Campbell

Animal Liberation
The Definitive Classic of the Animal Movement
Peter Singer

Why We Love Dogs, Eat Pigs, and Wear Cows
An Introduction to Carnism
Melanie Joy with foreword from John Robbins

Eat and Run
My Unlikely Journey to Ultramarathon Greatness
Scott Jurek with Steve Friedman

The Omnivore's Dilemma
A Natural History of Four Meals
Michael Pollan

Eating Animals
Groundbreaking Moral Examination of Vegetarianism, Farming, and the Food We Eat Every Day
Jonathan Safran Foer

We Are the Weather
Saving the Planet Begins at Breakfast
Jonathan Safran Foer

In Defence of Food
Don't Buy Food Where You'd Buy Your Petrol!
Michael Pollan

How to Create a Vegan World
A Pragmatic Approach
Tobias Leenaert

For A Moment of Taste
How What You Eat Impacts Animals, Planet and Earth
Poorva Joshipura

Animalkind
Remarkable Discoveries About Animals and Revolutionary New Ways to Show Them Compassion
Ingrid Newkirk, Gene Stone with foreword by Mayim Bialik

Meathooked
Our 2.5-Million-Year Obsession with Meat
Marta Zaraska

Farm to Fable
The Fictions of Our Animal-Consuming Culture
Robert Grillo

CHAPTER 51

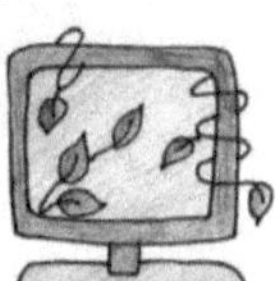

MUST-WATCH FILMS AND VIDEOS

Best Vegan Speech Ever
Gary Yourofsky on Worlds forgotten victims
1 Hrs, 13+, Gary Yourofsky's inspirational speech held at Georgia Tech in 2010 has changed the views of millions of people. A must watch.

Dominion
Produced by Actor, Joaquin Phoenix
2.0 Hrs, 13+, Exposing dark side of animal agriculture, questioning the humankind's dominion over the animal kingdom; from the producers of Earthlings.

Cowspiracy
Factory farming is decimating the environment
1.5 Hrs; 15+, Investigative, There are some graphic scenes of animal death.

End Game 2015
What will be the future be like in the year 2050, just 3 decades away.
1.5 Hrs; 13+, Investigative, Must watch.

The Game Changers
Sports and vegan food
2 Hrs, 16+, Produced by Arnold Schwarzenegger, Jackie Chan and others, Many sports and Olympic gold medalists are vegans; has few in-appropriate language.

Okja

On friendship between a girl and "super pig" Okja.
2 Hrs, 16+, In-appropriate language at places,

Supersize Me

Health risks of fast food and meat consumption
1.5 Hrs; 13+ PG, has some In-appropriate language and adult content,

Food inc

Meat industry, food business and questionable methods
1.5 Hrs; 13+ PG, Disturbing documentary. Teens and up.

Earthlings

The day-to-day practices of the largest industries in the world, all of which rely entirely on animals for profit.
1.5 Hrs, 18+, Horror, Extremely disturbing film, but must see

Forks Over Knives

Hard-to-deny evidence on obesity, diseases and meat
1.5 Hrs, 13+ PG , Engaging documentary promotes a vegan diet in nonjudgmental way. Scientific evidence mixed with personal stories

What the Health

Hidden dangers in the meat-eater's diet
1.5 Hrs, 13+, by the makers of Cowspiracy, Strong messages using scare tactics

Maximum Tolerated Dose

Heartbreaking stories on animal testing
1.5 Hrs, 16+, Lives of both humans and non-humans who have experienced animal testing first-hand, with hauntingly honest testimony of scientists

Live and Let Live
Relationship with animals and the history of veganism
1.5 Hrs, 13+, Stories of six individuals who decided to stop consuming animal products for different reasons

Called to Rescue
Every animal has a name and a story
1.0 Hr, 13+, Chance encounters, inner callings, and the unconditional love shared by animals are changing lives

The Cove
Man is their biggest threat and only hope
14+ PG, Gruesome, powerful, and inspiring Oscar-winning dolphin documentary, by Louie Psihoyos

Vegan: Everyday Stories
Lives of four remarkably different people
1.5 Hrs; 13+, Lives of four people who share a common thread, including a 8-year-old girl who convinces her family to go vegan

Vegucated
Lives of three meat-lovers who agree to go vegan
1 Hrs, 13+, Guerrilla-style documentary that follows three meat- and cheese-loving New Yorkers who agree to adopt a vegan diet for 6 weeks

A Prayer for Compassion
Can compassion grow to include all beings?
1.5 Hrs, 13+, Can people who identify as religious or spiritual come to embrace the call to include all human and nonhuman beings in our circle of respect, caring, and love?

The Big Fat Lie
Connection between food and diseases.
1.5 Hrs, 13+, How America's Plan for Eating Right Got It So Wrong

Racing Extinction
Biodiversity loss and species extinction
1.5 Hrs, 13+, About mass extinction of species and the efforts from scientists, activists and journalists - by Oscar-winning director Louie Psihoyos, who directed the documentary The Cove

Deadly Dairy
Deep dive into dairy
17 Mts. All around the world, people think Indians worship cows and don't torture them, but truth is different – by Animal Equality India

The Perils of Dairy
1 Hrs, Dairy is a great source of nutrition – for getting fat and growing tumors! – by John McDougall, MD

Speciesism: The Movie
Do not discriminated on the basis of species membership
1.5 Hrs. Documentary film by American director Mark Devries. It explores the concept and practice of speciesism, the assignment of value to beings on the basis of species membership

An Inconvenient Truth
Dangers of global warming
Produced by United States former Vice President Al Gore to to educate people about global warming.

Do search for these must-watch films in YouTube or Amazon Prime or Netflix or Vimeo. Check the movie ratings and reviews at IMDB, Common Sense Media, or Rotten Tomatoes and do watch with your family and friends to understand what is behind the food we eat. If you are pressed for time, we would suggest Best Vegan Speech Ever, Dominion and Game Changers.

CHAPTER 52

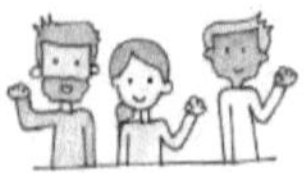

PEOPLE MAKING A DIFFERENCE

"If early in that year (1780s) you had stood on a London street corner and insisted that slavery was morally wrong and should be stopped, nine out of ten listeners would have laughed you off as a crack pot. The tenth might have agreed with you in principle but assured you that ending slavery was widely impractical." said Adam Hochschild, a historian (extract from book *A Plea for The Animals*).

Animal rights movement and vegan way of living are in the same state right now. There are many who are actively spearheading the cause of animal rights and vegan way of life, moving the mountains and human mindset.

"At first they ignore you, then laugh at you, then they fight you and then you win," said Mahatma Gandhi, which is equally applicable to the vegan movement and vegan awakening.

"When the number of those in favor of a new approach reaches a critical mass, public opinion begins to swing in their direction," says Matthiew Ricard.

Below is a quick illustrative list of people who are actively working for Animal rights and vegan way of life. This list is not exhaustive and for illustration purposes only. You can follow them on Instagram or Facebook or other social media to learn more and find your path to compassion, love and a vegan way of living.

Ed Winters (Earthling Ed)

Ed Winters is a vegan educator, public speaker and content creator based in London, England. His speech "You Will Never Look at Your Life in the Same Way Again" has over 33 million accumulative views online and has been given to thousands of students across UK universities.

W: https://earthlinged.org/
IG: @earthlinged
FB: earthlingedpage

Paul Bashir & Anonymous for the Voiceless

Paul Bashir along with Asal Alamdari run Anonymous for the Voiceless (AV), which is a grassroots animal rights organization specializing in street activism based in Australia. AV created the famous Cube of Truth activism, which is happening regularly all over the globe.

W: https://www.anonymousforthevoiceless.org/
IG: @anonymousforthevoiceless
FB: anonymousforthevoiceless

Hudson Tarlow

Hudson, 17 years old, has been involved with animal right activism. He organizes for AV Santa Monica and creates very impactful vegan activism on social media.

IG: @hudsontarlow
FB: hudsontarlowvegan
YT: Hudson Tarlow

Greta Thunberg

Greta Thunberg is a school-going Swedish environmental activist highlighting existential crisis arising from climate change. She is known for Fridays for the Future school strike moment. She is *Time*'s persona of the year and has been nominated for Nobel peace prize.

IG: @ gretathunberg
FB: gretathunbergsweden
YT : GretaThunberg

Natasha and Luca "That Vegan Couple"

After stressful careers, poor diets based on animal products, health problems, and desperately needing to change lives, Natasha and Luca became that vegan couple. They have a large following in social media.

W: https://thatvegancouple.com/
IG: @that_vegan_couple
FB: thatvegancouple
YT: movemevegan

Ana and Brian – Those Annoying Vegans

Ana and Brian, living in Los Angles, became vegans and vegan ambassadors to help others. They have a huge following in social media. They are vegan YouTubers and are changing hearts and minds of people one conversation at a time.

W: https://thatvegancouple.com/
IG: @ Thoseannoyingvegans
FB: Thoseannoyingvegans
YT: Those Annoying Vegans

Vegan Evan

Vegan Evan is a 9-year-old award-winning vegan activist and rapper. He is co-president and spokesperson for Animal Hero kids, a non-profit that reaches over 30,000 kids and teaches them kindness.

W: https://veganevan.com/
IG: @veganevan
FB: veganevan
YT: veganevan

Zoe Rosenberg / Zoe_Rooster

Zoe is a young American animal rights activist and the founder of Happy Hen Animal Sanctuary, a California-based sanctuary for abused and mistreated farmed animals. Zoe Rosenberg launched the "Meat-is-Immoral.com" campaign.

W: https://happyhen.org/
IG: @ zoe_rooster
FB: Zoe.Rooster

Ryuji

Ryuji (a film director), known as Peace by Vegan, produces exceptional activism content, which he mainly distributes through Instagram.

IG: @peacebyvegan
FB: peacebyvegan
YT : peacebyvegan

Amala Akkineni

Amala, a famous South Indian actress, animal lover, and founder of Blue Cross Hyderabad, India believes that veganism is the answer to end animal cruelty and to lead a healthy lifestyle

W: https://bluecrosshyd.org
IG: @ Akkineniamala
FB: Amala Akkineni

Maneka Gandhi

Maneka Gandhian, an Indian politician, animal rights activist, and environmentalist, has been promoting animal rights and a vegan way of living. When asked about food substitutes she said "you do not substitute poison with anything".

W: https://peopleforanimalsindia.org/
IG: @ pfa.offcial
FB: people4animals

Again, this list is not an exhaustive one. There are thousands of people working to create awareness on this important subject in all countries, including countries like India. I would encourage you to find people in your country, community, and people near you using social media, animal rights forums and vegan forums and connect with them.

"I like meat....I also like the feel of leather and fur. Nevertheless I no longer put animal products on my plate or on my shoulders. I no longer condone or overlook animal suffering. I am vegan.

It is not that I particularly like animals...
I am a normal type in my relationship to animals.
But I am also sensitive to moral arguments.
And today these arguments – with regard to animals and environmental ethics – have become too serious for me to set aside veganism with a shrug of the shoulder and wave of the hand.

Veganism is not a dietary program... It is a movement of resistance to the oppression of which the animals, we exploit for their meat, their milk or their fur, are the victims.

The basic argument is simple.
If it is possible to live without inflicting unnecessary suffering on animals, that is what we ought to do."

Martin Gibert
French Philosopher, Thinker, and Author
(as quoted in A Plea for Animals*)*

CHAPTER 53

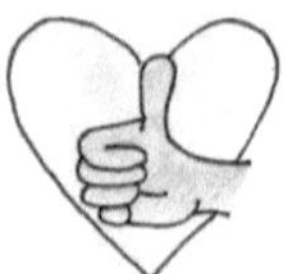

DO YOUR BIT TO HELP ANIMALS AND THIS MOVEMENT

We are working on possible ways to promote veganism, which helps in preventing cruelty to animals, reducing climate change and global warming, and making food and water available for everyone.

We all need to overcome the years of inertia and lethargy emanating from blind traditions, which do not make any sense now in the twenty first century and we need to overcome our addiction to meat and dairy.

Vegan or we're gone is published as a part of the efforts of **vegan4ever**, an organization working to spread awareness about vegan way of living.

We need to win over media and television advertisements that do such a good job in making animals look simply like a food product, like idli or dosa batter or a pack of semiya on supermarket shelves.

"Companies do an amazing job of hiding how animals spend most of their lives in cages, unable to move or turn around, or living knee-deep in their own shit and consuming antibiotics every day so that they do not fall ill," said Pandit Dasa, a vegan ambassador in the United

States. These businesses basically ride on the "but...I love my meat" addictiveness that we have inherited.

We need to educate people that "animals are friends and not food."

This idea is already resonating well with so many people around the world.

At vegan4ever.org, we plan to create awareness on animal rights and educate school students and college students on vegan way of living, by having sessions and distributing this book and other research materials.

We need your support in taking this ahimsa, non-violence, and vegan initiatives much wider and further, benefiting both animals and humans.

Please do strengthen the hands of vegans and vegan groups. Help the animals, our pre-existing co-travelers on planet Earth by becoming a vegan and helping others to go vegan.

Your decision can save so many lives.

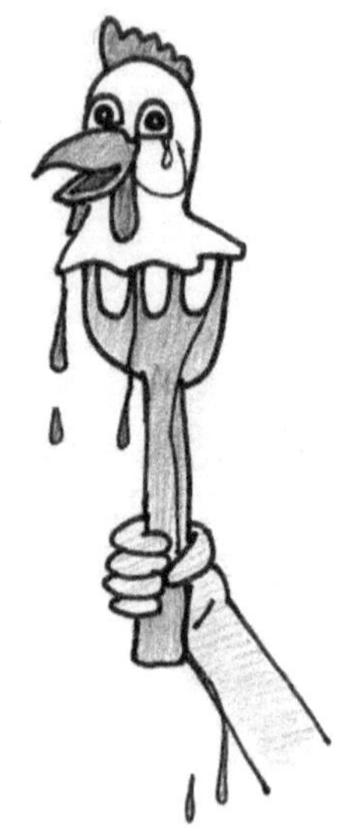

I can't decide what you
should eat,

Just like how
you can't decide when and
how an animal should die.

Manasa

ACKNOWLEDGMENTS

Thanks to my daughter Manasa, who opened my eyes and taught animals are "friends, not food."

She taught, repeatedly by her action, what it means to care for animals and being a vegan. I first learnt the meaning of the word vegan from her and understood it is about caring for animals and not a definition of food.

For my young son Manish, who at the prime age of 12, understood the concept of being vegan and had the guts as well as courage to kick those chocolates, ice creams, milkshakes, cheese pizzas, and biscuits out of his daily life, all in one go, saying "stop eating them is better than troubling, torturing, and slaughtering animals for food."

Tharangini, my wife, and I went vegan seeing my daughter and son go the vegan way. We used to be vegetarians but were consuming dairy almost all the day – for breakfast, lunch, and dinner and using dairy in the name of religion and culture. As a family, we went vegan for the sake of our co-travelers on earth, the animals.

Thanks to Gary Yourofsky for his "Best Speech You'll Ever Hear" video, which turned many to go vegan, including us.

Special thanks to Matthieu Ricard and his book *A Plea for Animals* which made me sit up, think, and write this small compilation. *A Plea for Animals* had a deep impact on me and improved my understanding of what is right, ethical, and good.

* * *

Thanks to Manasa, Manish, and Tharangini who contributed significantly to the contents of this book. They all ideally are co-authors of this book.

Big thanks to Aravind K from Tamil Vegans United, Chennai for his support in editing the book and his valuable suggestions.

* * *

Thanks to global media for recognizing raise of veganism. *The New York Times*, for example, wrote eye-opening articles including "Our Cruel Treatment of Animals Led to the Coronavirus" (April 13, 2020) and "End of Meat Is Here" (May 21, 2020). Other global media has been covering raise of veganism and its positive impact on earth and its co-travelers.

Thanks to growing number of thousands of vegans who are helping every one to see the unseen, shed light on "what goes behind the doors" at animal farms and slaughterhouses and eventually raising the human understanding and consciousness to the next level.

Special thanks to hundreds of vegan activists who are doing a great deal of work, globally, in each country and in each region.

Thanks to you – for taking time, reading and considering
how we all can change for better.

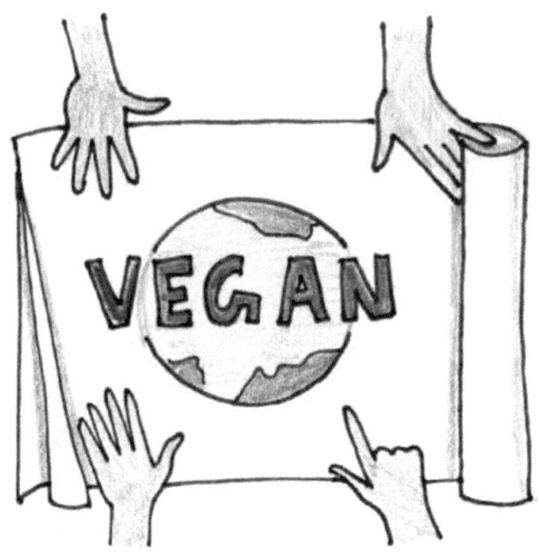

A brand-new vegan world is
unfolding in front of our eyes.

Which side of history you want to be
part of?

Veganism or
exploitation of animals and earth?